Arvid Kellgren

Technic of Ling's System of Manual Treatment

Arvid Kellgren

Technic of Ling's System of Manual Treatment

ISBN/EAN: 9783741122132

Manufactured in Europe, USA, Canada, Australia, Japa

Cover: Foto ©Lupo / pixelio.de

Manufactured and distributed by brebook publishing software
(www.brebook.com)

Arvid Kellgren

Technic of Ling's System of Manual Treatment

TECHNIC OF LING'S SYSTEM

OF

MANUAL TREATMENT

AS APPLICABLE TO

SURGERY AND MEDICINE.

BY

ARVID KELLGREN, M.D. (EDIN.).

REPRINTED FROM WOOD'S MEDICAL AND SURGICAL MONOGRAPHS.

NEW YORK:

WILLIAM WOOD & COMPANY.

1892.

CONTENTS.

CHAPTER VIII.

CHAPTER IX.

CHAPTER X.

CHAPTER XI.

CHAPTER XII.

CHAPTER XIII.

TECHNIC OF LING'S SYSTEM OF MANUAL TREATMENT.

CHAPTER I.

INTRODUCTION.

THE following pages are intended to serve as a guide to the student, and to set more clearly before the minds of readers the curative uses to which Ling's system of manual treatment may be applied. They mainly consist of sixteen demonstrations which were given by me at Pola during the winter of 1888–89. These lectures were delivered at the request of the surgeons of the Imperial and Royal Austro-Hungarian Navy, and also of the surgeons of the land forces stationed at Pola. Numerous illustrations have been added, in order to render more clear the directions in the text; and it is hoped that the work may prove not only of interest, but of practical utility, in the study of this form of medical treatment.

It is now more than eighty years since the idea of curing diseases by well-regulated movements first occurred to the Swede, Peter Henrik Ling.

P. He. Ling was born in the year 1776. His father was a Protestant minister. He went through the usual course of training preparatory to entering the university, where, in accordance with his parents' desire, he took up the study of divinity. The tendency of Ling's character, however, disposed him to a more active life, and as soon as he was free to follow his own inclinations, he started travelling on the Continent.

Very little is known about him during his wanderings. Certain it is that he returned home well versed in foreign languages, and a perfect master of the art of fencing; but also, in consequence of the hardships he had undergone, with a shattered constitution. This, however, did not prevent him from following his favorite pursuits, and we thus find him at the beginning of the century working hard at gymnastics and fencing.

Ling gradually regained his health, and on his appointment, in 1804, to the post of fencing master at the University of Lund, he was a strong and wiry man. He rightly attributed the change to the gymnastic exercises he had taken; and he further drew the conclusion that what had been good for him would also be good for others, and that it ought to be possible to devise movements which would be particularly beneficial for invalids.

He was a man of indomitable energy, the whole of which he brought to bear on the carrying out of these plans. The professors of medicine at the University of Lund were friends of his, and he endeavored to interest them in his ideas, and succeeded to a certain extent in so doing. They opened their anatomy and other lecture-rooms to him, and helped him in many ways. The "fencing master," as some of the continental writers on massage, the majority of whom know nothing whatever of his treatment, are so fond of calling him, learned everything that could in those days be learned in the different departments of medical study.

By utilizing and developing many of the gymnastic movements practised by former men, and by devising for himself many new ones, he built up a system of exercises—the Ling system. He studied their effect, and endeavored to explain it on physiological grounds. As we cannot always explain the action of many drugs, so he was unable to explain why certain exercises produced corresponding results. He was in these cases guided by the law of the beautiful, and reasoned that any exercise or movement which in itself was graceful, would also be beneficial.

He divided his system into four chief branches:

1. The pedagogic.
2. The medical.
3. The military.
4. The æsthetic.

I only intend in this thesis to deal more particularly with the second group, but I may say that the "pedagogic" exercises are for the developing and strengthening of healthy people, while the "medical" are meant to arrest or combat diseased conditions.

These two, however, pass so gradually into one another that no distinct line can be drawn between them; and it is therefore essential to know both, in order to be able to use the medical part of the system properly for the purpose assigned to it.

Being anxious to found a gymnastic institution, Ling applied for help to the government, but the Minister of State to whom he addressed himself replied, "We have enough of jugglers and dancers on wires without also subsidizing them by the state." But in the year 1812 his efforts were crowned with success, and the government of Sweden founded "The Royal Central Gymnastic Institution" in Stockholm, with Ling as its chief.

Here regular courses of lectures on anatomy and physiology were given, the pedagogic and medical gymnastics taught, together with fencing in all its branches. No pupil was allowed to enter the institution who had not passed the university entrance examination, which corresponds to the "Abiturienten Examen" in Germany. At the present time a nine-months' course of instruction is given each year, viz., from the 1st September to the 15th of May.

When Ling died, on the 3d of May, 1839, he left to his country, that numbers him among her greatest sons, in the form of his system of exercises, a legacy by which thousands have regained their health, and by which, thanks to the pedagogic portion, there still lives in Sweden a strong and healthy people.

The path, however, of this new method was not a smooth one, for so soon as the effect of the treatment began to show itself, the Swedish medical profession did everything in their power to prevent its further progress. At first they tried to kill the system by silence or assailed it with sarcasm, but finding these means useless, in the face of cures resulting from its application, they began an active resistance.

Those, however, who advocated the system—and among them, proving exceptions to the general rule, were several medical men—were by far too enthusiastic in favor of the treatment to be easily frightened from what they considered the right path.

When I spent the years 1877–79 in the institution, only a two-years' course was necessary in order to obtain a diploma, but in the year 1888 the rule was made that a three-years' course should be imperative. The concluding year is entirely devoted to attendance at lectures on diseases, to clinics, and to the application of the various movements to the patients undergoing treatment. The latter are of two classes—those in the morning being paying patients, while in the afternoon the poor are gratuitously treated. This valuable and necessary extension of time is due to the present chief of the institution, Professor L. M. Torngren, Professor Hartelius, and the other masters, who for over six years have strenuously advocated the acceptance of this rule by the Swedish Medical Council.

It is supposed by many that what nowadays goes under the name of massage is one thing and Ling's system is another. This is an entire mistake, for the massage manipulations are only a few of the passive movements contained in Ling's system. That this is the case, any one may see for himself, if he will read what Ling and his immediate successors have written. It is, on the other hand, quite true that the medical profession in Sweden, disregarding their own native institution, have "gone over the river to fetch water," and have learnt the massage movement from Metzger or his pupils.

I should also wish to state that I have not studied any part of the treatment under any one but my own masters in the Royal Central Institution at Stockholm, and my brother, Mr. Henrik Kellgren, under whom I worked more or less during the years 1876 to 1886. Neither have I read all the writings on massage and Ling's system ("Schwedische Heilgymnastik") which are everywhere cropping up on the Continent. But the little of these authors that I have read, and the figures I have seen in their books purporting to be true illustrations of Ling's exercises, are in most cases incorrect.

Another impression derived from these books is, that the authors, if they have ever been in Stockholm, must have been there during the summer, when the institution is closed, or at any rate have stayed there too short a time to learn anything.

Let me also state, that part of what I describe—*i.e.*, most of the shakings, nearly all the vibrations and the nerve vibrations—are not part of Ling's original system, but have been added by my brother, Mr. Henrik Kellgren, who was a pupil under Ling junior.

It is hardly necessary to add, that we who advocate Ling's system such as he taught it, do not use any machines for producing the movements. We certainly have apparatus, if I may so call it, on or beside which the patient may take up certain positions which enable us to give the exercises where we wish, and as we wish. Machines cannot possibly do the work of the human hand, which has the brain controlling it. If the machine could feel and think, it might be otherwise. The condition of the patient varies from day to day, and so must the treatment. This can be readily done when we use our hands, but not when machines are employed. Professor Branting, the greatest of all the pupils of Ling senior, speaking of the machines, said, "De representera hedendomen i gymnastiken"—"they represent the heathen times of the treatment." I readily admit it is more comfortable to do the work with the machines, but as the patient should be our first consideration, I have no hesitation in saying that no machines will produce results comparable with manual exercises properly applied.

It is generally considered that the manual treatment is quiet inapplicable for acute inflammation of the joints and other parts. This commonly entertained belief is a complete mistake. Certainly, if we rely only on the ordinary massage movements in these acute conditions, we can do little good, and probably will do harm; but in vibrations and nerve frictions, we possess a strong weapon with which to combat these acute diseases. The difficulty lies in the application of these vibrations, for if they are given with an unskilled hand, the effect is frequently not beneficial; but this fact can scarcely be quoted as an argument against their use, or the treatment itself. Among the cases which I append, it will be found that I mention examples of acute inflammation, such as diphtheria, tonsillitis, parotitis, recent fractures, etc., which were treated at once.

In giving the massage manipulations, I never use oil or ointment of any kind. The dry massage is cleaner, it affords a better and more certain feeling to the hand, the movements are steadier, and it is seldom necessary to expose the patient's body, except occasionally for purposes of examination. For example, in pétrissage of the abdomen, a linen or silk garment intervenes between the hand of the manipulator and the skin of the patient.

It should be added that mere theoretical teaching will never train any one to give the exercises properly. To gain complete mastery of the movements necessitates several years of careful work, as seen from the fact that the course at Stockholm has been extended to three years. Moreover, a special aptitude is required for the treatment, which even long experience will not create—just as one man may bring to the practice of operative surgery a neatness and dexterity of handling which others may work for years without being able to acquire. The treatment, in short, is one that cannot lightly be taken up in connection with other forms of medical work, but should either be exclusively practised or left alone.

The medical part of Ling's system is divided into

I. Passive Movements.

A passive movement is one which is executed on the patient, or with a part of him, he himself being entirely at rest.

The passive movements are as follows:

1. Effleurage.
2. Pétrissage.
3. Tapotement.
4. Massage à friction.
5. Rolling and shaking of the muscles.
6. Shakings.
7. Vibrations.
8. Nerve vibrations.
9. Passive extension of muscles.
10. Other passive movements, such as rolling, extension and flexion, etc., at the different joints.

II. Active Movements.

A movement is called active when the patient himself takes a working part in it.

The active movements are divided into—

1. Free, *i.e.*, movements executed by the patient without any external help whatever.

2. Bound, *i.e.*, movements made either while steadiness and isolation are secured by apparatus, or under resistance.

Those made under resistance are again subdivided into—

(α) Those in which the patient resists.

(β) Those in which the operator resists.

CHAPTER II.

PASSIVE MOVEMENTS.

THROUGH the passive movements we act more or less directly on the part or organ which is to be subjected to treatment. Acting more particularly on the venous and lymphatic circulation, they must all be made in the direction of those currents. They all have a common physiological effect, viz., of causing resorption.

Some of the passive exercises which are executed with a part of the patient's body, approach in their character the active movements—as, for instance, the rolling of a limb, such as the arm, when we quickly rotate it at the shoulder-joint.

EFFLEURAGE.

Effleurage is a stroking movement in the direction of the heart, the object being to act more particularly on the venous and lymphatic circulation in superficial parts, such as the skin, subcutaneous tissues, etc.

The effleurage may be very superficial or deep—in other words, the pressure may vary from the lightest touch to one of considerable force; but this force must be gradually increasing as it passes toward freer and healthier parts, and should not be applied with vigor from the outset.

The superficial form of effleurage is intended to soothe pain by its action on the endings of the sensory nerves in the skin, while the deeper has for its purpose the onward passage of fluids. In any case, both forms must, according to my opinion, be made slowly. If the hand is passed quickly over the skin, heat and redness of the surface are caused. The operator has thus produced hyperæmia of the skin, i.e., drawn the blood to the distal side say of an effusion—and that is

certainly a very questionable advantage. Besides, in the deep
effleurage it gives the patient more pain.

If the effleurage is only superficial, one ought to begin at
the extremity of the limb; when it is deep, however, a commencement should be made somewhat higher than the upper
border of the swelling.

Take, for instance, effleurage of the right forearm when
effusions are present (Fig. 1).

The patient rests his arm on a table, and the operator
steadies it still more by grasping the wrist with his left hand.
He then, with the radial border of his right hand forward,
makes a stroking movement from below upward, beginning at

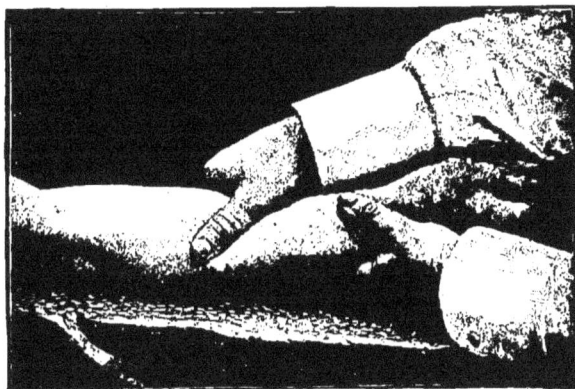

FIG. 1.

first above the effusion and gradually coming down, allowing
each individual stroke to have its normal direction.

The effleurage ought to begin higher up than the exudation
extends, in order to stimulate the tissues above to brisker
activity, and it must be carried step by step downward,
because the amount of exudation which is driven forward is
of course far less than it would be if one started at the extremity of the limb. The consequence of this, again, is, that
more force can be used, less pain is caused to the patient, and
the resorption is quicker.

The operator should be careful to hold his own arm as
nearly as possible parallel to that of the patient. The manipulation is thus easier to give, and is less hard, as every bending
in the wrist-joint causes more stiffness in it, greater pressure

on the part worked on, and also changes the direction of the force.

The part of the hand with which to work depends on the portion of the body to be acted on, and the cause. For instance, round the ankle, or for thickening of a tendon, the first phalanx of the thumb or the fingers is used, but not in such a pointed manner as is generally shown in diagrams.

For my own part, I never give effleurage first, but invariably precede it with some other movement, such, for example, as pétrissage. Most operators, on the contrary, usually begin with it. There are, I understand, even those who, as a preparation, for several days limit their treatment to this movement alone, and that only round the affected part, if it be painful, as in a distortion. That is to say, the exudation is allowed to settle, and the pain caused by it at the beginning is not relieved. Such a procedure is simply a waste of time. I have given pétrissage and effleurage at once in fresh distortions, dislocations, fractures of the fibula, radius, and round the elbow, and I have never had the slightest reason to regret this method.

To give effleurage for neuralgic pains is a still greater error, because there are other easier and more effective manipulations suited to the cure—I mean nerve vibrations.

Whenever effleurage is given in any affection where the slightest movement produces pain, one hand must be used to steady the part. In fact, I invariably make it a rule to do this even when there is no pain. It gives me greater command over the limb, and the manipulation is more accurate.

I have seen diagrams showing effleurage of the throat. There has been, according to my judgment, one common mistake in them, viz., the leaning back of the head. The movement, I suppose, is to have its effect by the centripetal pressure produced on the vena jugularis interna. But if we look at the anatomical arrangement of the parts, we shall find that the sterno-cleido-mastoid and omohyoid muscles cross the vein, and must also produce their pressure when the head is thrown back. If anything is to be avoided it is decidedly positions which in themselves hinder the venous circulation—much more so then, when, as in the present case, they are entirely unnecessary, since the completely erect position is the correct one.

As regards the duration of effleurage, this depends on the cause of treatment. I am quite unable to offer an opinion as to how long effleurage should be given in order to lull pain alone, because I always use nerve vibrations. Under other circumstances, 1 prefer a few slow, strong, and deep strokes to any number of light and quick ones.

CHAPTER III.

PÉTRISSAGE.

PÉTRISSAGE is a kneading movement, by which the skin, subcutaneous tissues, and more particularly muscles, are acted upon.

The muscle, or part of it, is grasped slowly between the thumb and the other fingers, and rolled slowly between them, in very much the same manner as one rolls a pencil, the pressure sometimes increasing, sometimes diminishing, care being taken that the joints of the fingers and wrist are kept loose. A stiff wrist impedes the free motion of the fingers, and excludes the elasticity in them.

It is of importance in all forms of pétrissage, that the skin under the fingers should move with them, as the manipulation otherwise is somewhat uncertain and less effective. If we treat, for instance, such cases as erysipelas and frost-bite, and allow the fingers to move on the surface of the skin, these complaints are greatly intensified; while, when the manipulations are made correctly, the patients quickly recover. A short time ago I was called to a patient, a lady about thirty-eight years old, whose left ear had been attacked by erysipelas. She had felt somewhat feverish for a few days, and on the night preceding my call the illness had broken out. The ear was greatly swollen, the skin felt hard, tense, and infiltrated, and had an intensely red coloration; pain was present, and it increased on touch. The swelling and redness extended down on the throat for about two inches, and forward over the parotid region of the face; the lymphatic glands on the left side of the throat were enlarged. Fever and headache were also present.

Locally, I gave mostly pétrissage, in addition to some general treatment for the head and body. After two days the ear had its normal color and proportions, the skin peeled off, and the swelling on the face and neck were gone. For some days afterward the patient had a feeling of prickling and slight heat when the face and ear were washed.

The masseur can easily know if he has broken through the rule of not working with a stiff wrist and fingers, if the skin

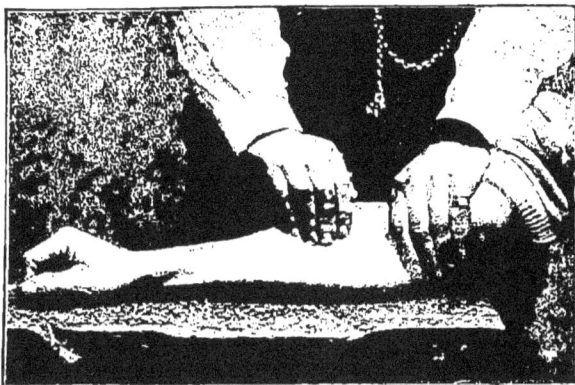

FIG. 2.

has been reddened more than from ordinary pressure, the redness of the latter being less intense, and disappearing more quickly. It seems scarcely necessary to state that the

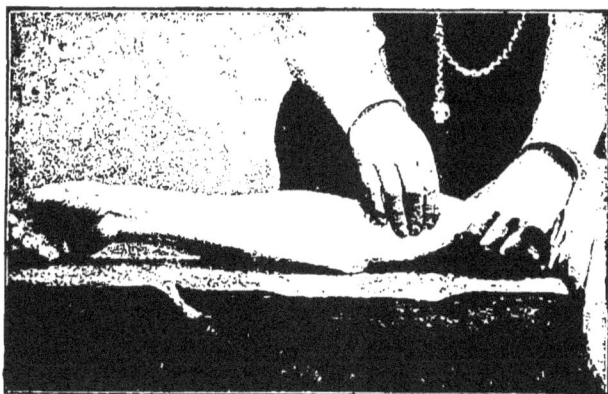

FIG. 3.

pressure should gradually increase in strength, but, as I have frequently seen mistakes of this kind made, I mention it.

The pétrissage to the muscles may be applied with one or with two hands, as shown in Figs. 2 and 3.

2

The manipulation with one hand hardly needs any further explanation, but with two hands it is more complicated. The muscle is rolled as before described, but it is also stretched by the backward movement of the fingers of one hand, while the thumb of the other passes forward. In Fig. 3 we also see that at the conclusion of the movement, the fingers of the hand moving forward and the thumb of the other one are only lightly in contact with the skin, and do not exert any pressure. If they did, we should have a constant pressure, less stretching of the muscle, and the stream of the fluids in the muscle would be interrupted; while, in addition, the skin would be strained in a way that would be very uncomfortable for the

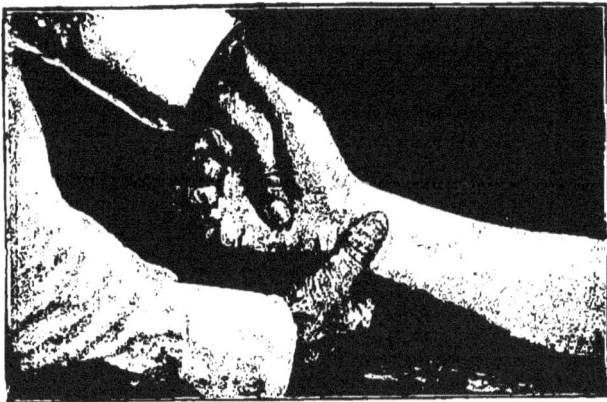

FIG. 4

patient. Care must be taken that the very tips of the fingers are not used, but at least the last phalanx as a whole and the anterior part of the second one as well. The use of the tips of the fingers and the thumb has been one of the commonest faults I have met with. One cannot work with the tips without strongly bending the fingers, which has the effect of stiffening them and the wrist. The softness in the movement becomes lost, the patient strains and contracts the muscle from the pain produced (e.g., in rheumatism, and even if there is no acute disorder), and the work becomes only superficial.

In giving pétrissage of a muscle, we ought always to begin at its proximal end, and gradually pass downward. Here, as in effleurage, we must take care, that each kneading has a

direction upward. This is easily produced by a slight twisting
of the hand.

When effusions arising from sprains, dislocations, or fractures are treated with pétrissage, I work with the whole of
the thumb down to its thenar part. I start above the effusion.

In order to obtain a larger and freer range of motion, the
thumb is put down a little above the place to be subjected to
manipulation, and carried back to the particular area to be
treated. If this precaution is not taken, the skin becomes
stretched and irritated by the onward movement of the thumb.
The thumb describes a half circle, with gradually increasing
pressure as long as it moves in the centripetal direction, then

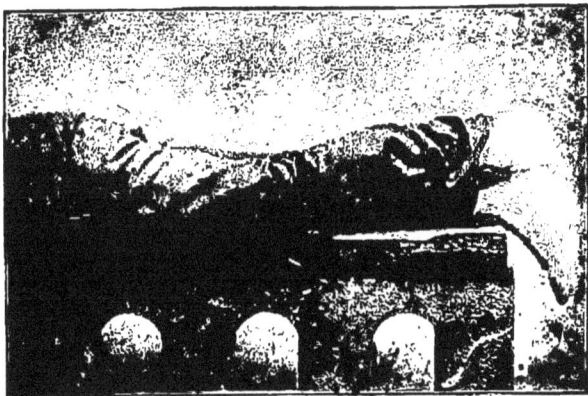

FIG. 5.

the pressure is relaxed, the thumb is lightly moved back to
the starting-place, and the same action repeated. The movement should be given slowly and deliberately.

In the gluteal region the manipulation is made with the
lightly-closed hand, and has the direction toward the sacrum.
The patient can then bear the treatment much easier, and will
allow it to go deeper.

The patient must always be placed in such a position that
the muscles to be worked at are relaxed. Thus, in pétrissage
for the gluteal region, he lies face downward, with the leg of
the affected side crossed over the other, as in Fig. 5. He is
not to stand bent forward, as is sometimes shown in illustrations, because the muscles are then more or less passively

extended, and prevent the proper application of the treatment.

In cases of incomplete fracture, or when the exudation is too great, gentle pétrissage with the first phalanx of the thumb enables one to come down to the seat of the injury, and thus aids to form a correct diagnosis.

When I treat effusion by pétrissage, I either pass over the whole of it two or three times, afterward making some strokes of deep effleurage, or I make one single stroke each time before moving the hand lower down.

The length of time to give pétrissage must of course vary with the case we are treating, it being necessary to apply it for some time in effusions and more serious complaints, while for simple stimulation of the muscles only a few minutes are necessary.

GENERAL PÉTRISSAGE OF THE ABDOMEN.

The position in which general or partial pétrissage of the abdomen is to be administered to the patient, is the recumbent

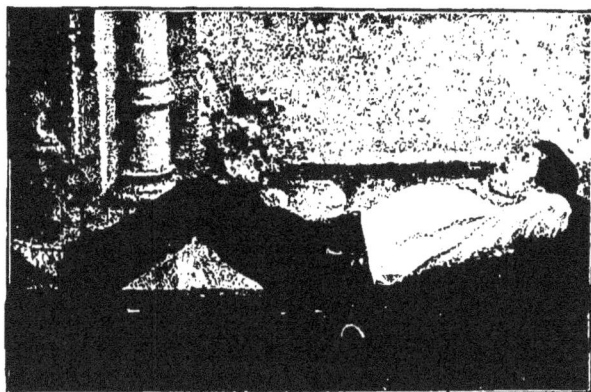

FIG. 6.

one shown in Fig. 6. It has for its object the relaxation of the abdominal muscles. The hands are folded behind the neck, in order to promote freer respiration. The patient is not allowed to lift the head up, because then the abdominal muscles at once contract, as any one may see for himself by lying down and raising the head. This result is very natural. The muscles which lift the head have their steady attachment on the thorax, and in order that this may be able to act as a point of leverage, it must itself be steadied by the abdominal muscles.

In general pétrissage of the abdomen, the whole of the palmar surface of the hand is in contact with the abdominal wall. The hand is spread out over it, the fingers lying to the left in the interval between the lower ribs and the iliac crest, but somewhat nearer the former, while the thumb has the same position on the right side, and the base of the hand is a little above the pubic arch, with the strongest part, the ball of the thumb, near the right iliac fossa.

As this manipulation and others of the abdomen are never

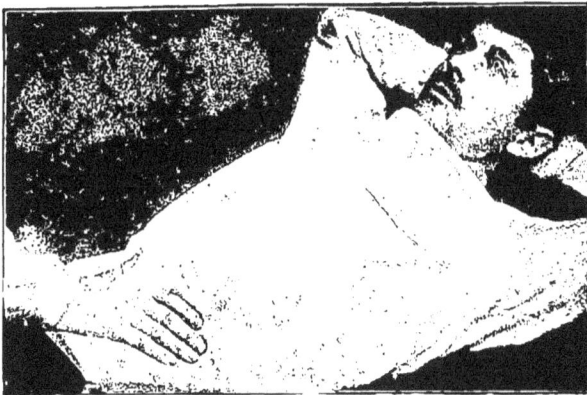

FIG. 7.

given on the bare body, it is of the highest importance that the part of the abdominal wall under the hand should follow it in its movements, otherwise irritation of the skin is caused. In order to decrease the possibility of this, the dress nearest to the skin ought not to consist of wool, but should be made of silk or linen. It is also clear that if the hand moves over the surface of the abdomen, the intestines are not acted upon, or only very slightly. It is of the utmost importance that the hand works firmly and yet softly, that there is no stiffness in any joint, and that the forearm is kept as nearly as possible parallel to the patient's body.

The movement itself has a circular character, and is generally started from below with the base of the hand. This, with slight extension (dorsal flexion) at the wrist, passes under soft, gradually-increasing pressure to the right into the iliac fossa, and then upward in the line of the ascending colon. It is natural that the thumb is brought higher up and comes to lie close under the ribs over the hepatic flexure. The hand now moves, always in contact with the abdominal wall, and continuing its slightly circular way to the left, the thumb and the thenar part of the hand having overtaken the work. It is not enough to move the hand over; it is also pronated a little at the same time, and the thumb is adducted toward the fingers. These again, as the hand passes to the left, come over the splenic flexure, and in their turn become the principal agents. They move downward, bending more and more at the metacarpo-phalangeal joints, not at the phalangeal ones, and with a slight flexion at the wrist. As the hand passes lower and lower down close beside the os ilium, it is somewhat supinated, and when the wrist is again near the pubic arch, the base of the hand again takes up the work.

These manipulations, although described separately, do not exactly follow each other, but one begins a little before the other has ended, and in this manner the kneading is produced. If this were not done, there would, of course, only be pressure in one direction after the other.

From the wide extent of the movement, we see that the whole of the intestine becomes rolled and kneaded, the circulatory activity is increased, and this carries with it increased absorption and secretion, and also increased peristaltic action of the intestine. We can also understand that it must have a great influence on the circulation in general, because of the large number of blood-vessels contained in the abdomen.

I have described this general pétrissage of the abdomen as practised by my brother, Mr. Henrik Kellgren. He nearly always gives it for some minutes, as the final movement of a day's treatment, because he has found that it greatly increases the quickness of recovery. The movement is very difficult, and, indeed, nearly impossible to describe well, but is also as difficult and as impossible to give for any one who has not been gifted by nature with a good hand for the treatment, and it is necessary both to see and still more to feel it.

It is tiresome at first for beginners, or when given often, and the fatigue is especially felt in the small muscles of the thumb. Much relief, however, may be derived by placing the fingers of the left hand on the thumb in such a manner that the tip of the long finger is over the phalangeal joint, and those of the fore and ring fingers respectively on the first and second phalanx.

Nearly all the organs in the abdominal cavity may separately come in for treatment. I will only describe special pétrissage for the colon and rectum, the kidneys, and above the pubic arch.

For the Colon and Rectum.

Pétrissage is here mostly given for constipation. There are especially two places to which our attention must be

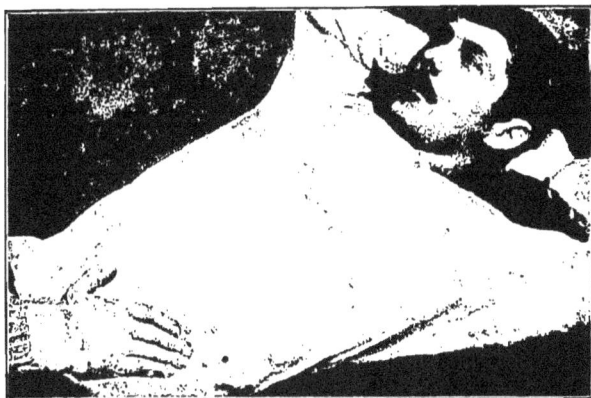

FIG. 8.

directed, viz., the sigmoid flexure of the colon and the splenic flexure of the colon. We begin the movement as far down in the pelvis as possible, and gradually pass upward. Each individual kneading always goes from above downward in the line of the intestine. The fingers are to be flexed only at the metacarpo-phalangeal joint, because if the fingers are bent the manipulation becomes pointed and painful, we cannot get down deep enough, and the kneading character is lost. As illustrative of this treatment, I may mention a case of constipation in a baby between three and four weeks old, which I had under my care while staying with a friend in Sweden last autumn. For two days medical applications had been tried, when I suggested to my friend, that his baby would not get well until I had given it some pétrissage of the abdomen. He gave me a look that clearly indicated that he was not likely to allow me to try anything of that kind. As the baby's condition on the third evening had not changed for the better, and all the medical resources at my friend's disposal, down to soap suppositories, were at an end, his aversion to my proposal passed away, and he even asked me to do what I could. I simply gave light pétrissage of the descending colon for about one minute, without the child making the slightest sound; but I dare say it would have been different, if I had bent my fingers and worked more with their tips. The bowels acted very well during the night, and no further treatment was necessary.

The left hand is often used to support the right, and then the tips of its fingers are placed on the last phalangeal joint, and its palmar surface close to the back of the right hand.

For the Kidneys.

We generally treat both at the same time. The abdominal wall must be very relaxed, as we need to bring the hand deep down before the manipulation can be begun.

The knees are bent somewhat more than in Fig. 6. The

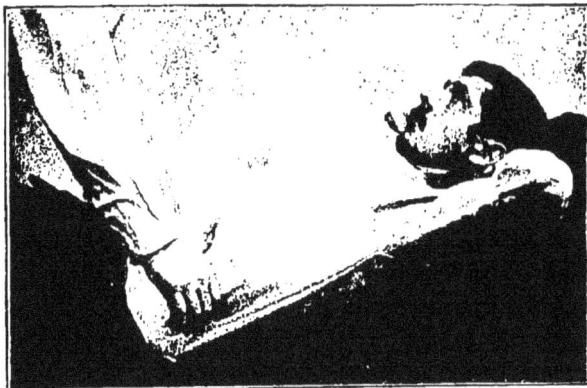

Fig. 9.

thumbs are placed and kept steady on the abdominal wall, on places corresponding to the situations of the kidneys, just below the ribs; and the patient is told to breathe very deeply.

As he now makes strong expirations, we come further and further down, until we can at least easily feel the kidneys. Then the patient has to make thoracic respiration, so that the manipulation may not be hindered by the movement of the abdominal muscles. The kneading is made from without inward, and slightly from above downward, in order that the pressure may be applied in the direction of the venous circulation and the larger number of the renal canals. One kidney may be treated at a time. We then use the palmar surface of the fingers, and, while giving the treatment, stand or sit on the opposite side to the kidney subjected to manipulation.

ABOVE THE PUBIC ARCH.

In pétrissage above the pubic arch, the hand is placed just above it, and is spread out in a manner similar to that in general pétrissage of the abdomen. The movement here goes from side to side, and the kneading is made with the fingers and the root of the hand.

CHAPTER IV

TAPOTEMENT means hacking or beating. The muscles principally in action are sometimes the flexors and extensors of the hand (palmar and dorsal); sometimes the radial and ulnar flexors. There is movement at the elbow. The joints of the wrist and hands are to be kept loose, no matter what kind of tapotement is given. This renders the manipulation

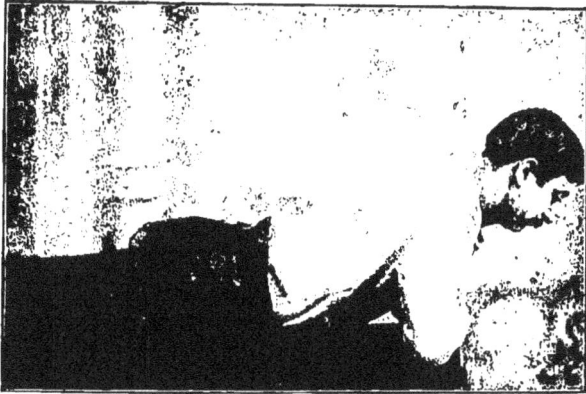

FIG. 10.

less hard and more elastic; the hand is heavier, and thus the effect of the stroke goes deeper.

The position of the hand, and the part of it which comes in contact with the body, must vary with the regions operated on.

The positions in which the patients are placed for the more advantageous application of this manipulation are generally:

For the Back.—The patient may lie face downward (as in Fig. 10), when frictions over the sensory nerves precede the manipulation, or he stands up slightly bending forward, with

his hands steadied, say against a wall. In both positions it is
necessary to see that the chest is not compressed by a too
near approximation of the arms to each other. They are
never to be nearer than the transverse diameter of the thorax.

For the Liver.—The patient either has the hands folded
behind his neck, as in Fig. 11, or with the right arm stretched
up, as in Fig. 28.

For the Lumbar Region.—The positions are the same as
for the back. We may also give the tapotement while the

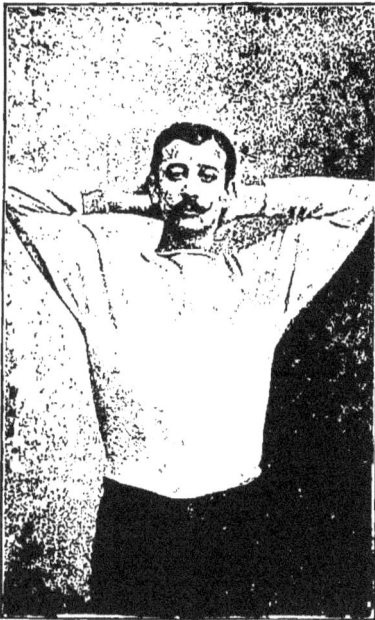

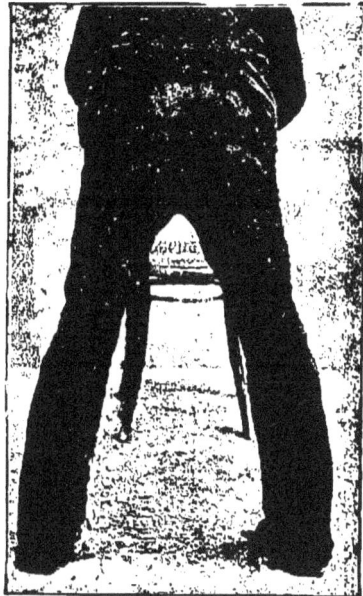

FIG. 11.   FIG. 12.

patient, with extended arms (upward), bends forward or sideways.

For the Sacral, Gluteal, and Perineal Regions.—The
patient takes up the position shown in Fig. 12; or the beating
is given in connection with the active movement shown in Fig.
56.

At the different parts of the body the tapotement is given
as follows:

On the Head.—Tapotement is made with the ulnar side of
the fingers, or with their tips; but this procedure is entirely

unnecessary, and nerve vibrations and frictions should be used instead.

On the Chest.—The palm of the hand is used (Fig. 13).

We see that the right hand, which is about to make the stroke, is not kept straight. It is only straightened out at the last moment, partly by a slight action of the extensor muscles, partly by the swing of the stroke. The difference between the stroke of a hand with fingers straight and the wrist stiff, and one held as I have just described, is indeed great. In the

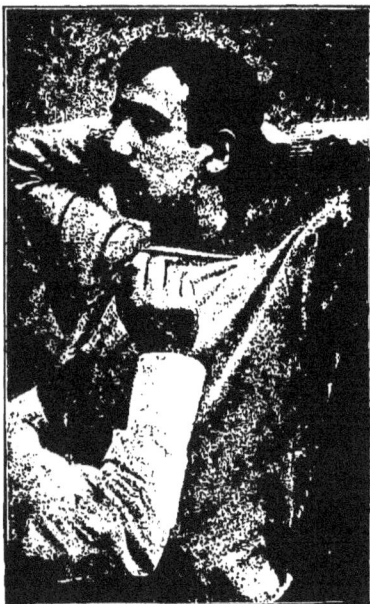

FIG. 13.

former case, the weight of the hand falling on the chest is lessened, and the effect is more external than internal, where it is expected to set the air into vibration, and stimulate the lungs.

The operator stands in front of the patient, and passes the arms round his chest until the hands have come well up between the shoulder-blades of the patient. He now begins the beating, passing up and down between the shoulder-blades, then over the sides of thorax, and lastly the front of the chest is treated. The patient makes deep and slow inspirations all the time.

It is given in chronic affections of the lungs, and is accompanied by movements which produce deep respiration.

On the Back.—The hands are kept midway between supination and pronation, with the fingers slightly bent (Fig. 14).

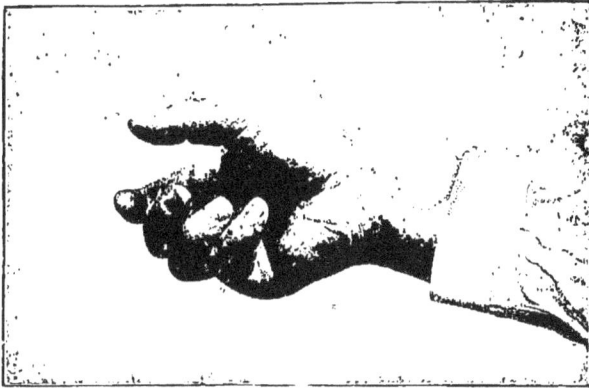

FIG. 14.

Just before the hand strikes the back it is more supined, in order that the ulnar edge itself may not strike, but that part

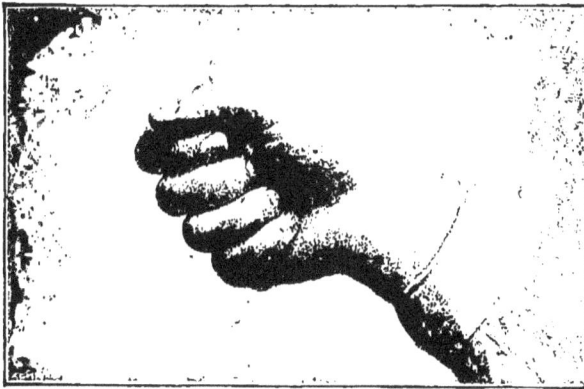

FIG. 15.

of the dorsal surface of the hand which is just outside it. The advantages of this are a softer blow, the fingers are spread out more, and deeper and superficial tissues are thus stimulated at the same time.

The movement should be carried three or four times up and down the back, parallel to and a little to the side of the vertebral column.

On the Lumbar Region.—We pass transversely over it, in order to be able to apply the treatment more powerfully, as the muscular mass is greater.

For the Liver.—The hacking is made over the lower part of the right side of the thorax, with the hand held in the same manner as for the back.

For the Sacral, Gluteal, and Perineal Regions, we keep the hands closed, but not firmly so. The stroke in the first

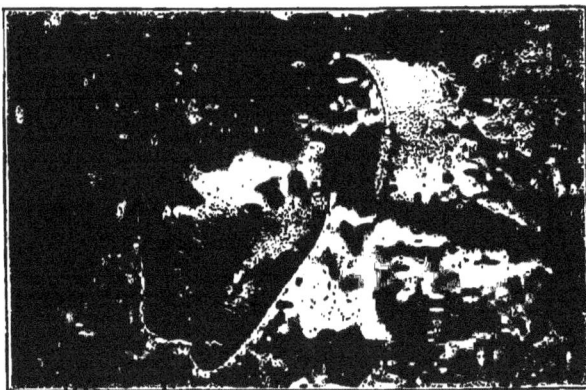

FIG. 16.

two cases is applied with the anterior part of the closed hand (Fig. 15); in the last, with the radial side (Fig. 16), because otherwise it cannot well enter the perineal space.

Tapotement in these places is made in connection with the treatment of constipation, disorders of the bladder, male and female generative organs.

For the Limbs.—The hands are either held in the same way as for the back, or the radial sides of the two hands are worked with simultaneously. The fingers are not to be kept extended, but loosely flexed, as in Fig. 17.

Whenever tapotement is given, stroke must follow upon stroke in quick succession, in order to increase the intensity of the manipulation.

The tapotement sets the muscular fibres into vibration, and

stimulates them to contract, the activity in superficial vessels and nerves is increased, and, as said before, when applied to

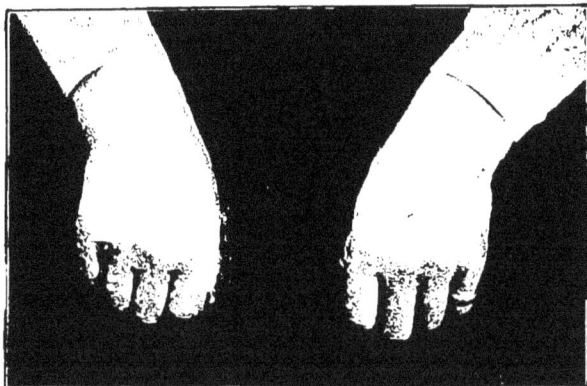

FIG. 17.

the back and thorax, the vibration is propagated on to internal parts. The duration of the manipulation is of necessity everywhere very short.

CHAPTER V.

MASSAGE À FRICTION.

FOR my own part, I cannot see the use of this expression, as the movement is certainly a kneading one, and thus only a modification of pétrissage.

The movement is the same as pétrissage, with the thumb alone, or with one or more of the fingers, but they are put at a greater—generally right—angle toward the part worked

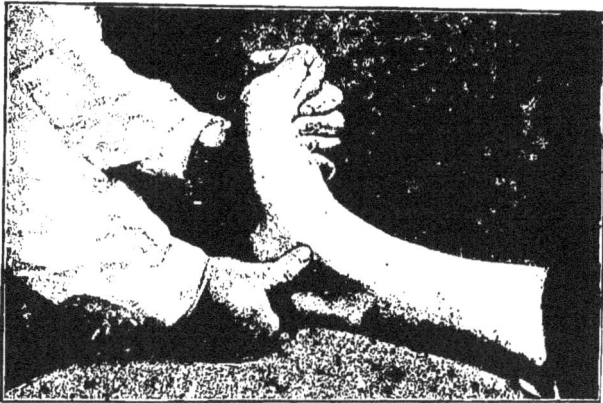

FIG. 18.

upon (Fig. 18); the circular or elliptical movement is smaller, and the pressure more equal throughout, as we wish simply by mechanical force to reduce thickenings and depositions. Effleurage follows on it, or is given alternately with the friction.

Massage à friction is chiefly had recourse to for organized exudations or hardened depositions, which we find round joints, such as the ankle, wrist, knee, etc., and for thickening of tendons.

CHAPTER VI.

GENERAL ROLLING AND SHAKING OF THE MUSCLES OF THE EXTREMITIES.

THE rolling and the shaking can easily be made at the same time on the limbs. The muscles must be completely relaxed. Take, for instance, the arm. The patient holds it in a horizontal position by steadying the hand on a table or the back of a chair. Both hands of the operator are placed lightly

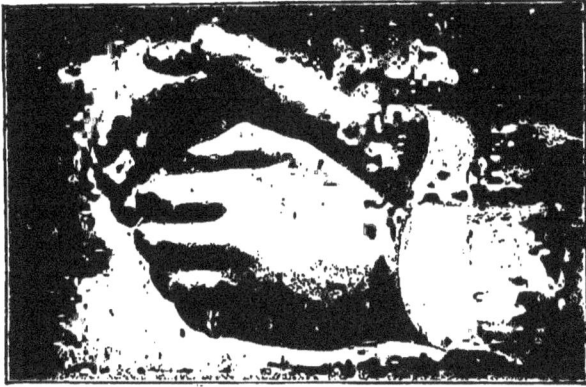

on the arm, and are moved quickly round it as they pass up and down two or three times (Fig. 19).

The effect is very stimulating and agreeable to the patient.

This manipulation should be used after pétrissage, but may also be given alone in cases where there is no cause for a more special treatment of any particular muscle.

3

CHAPTER VII.

SHAKING.

THE part of the hand which, during the manipulation of shaking, comes in contact with the patient's body, is the distal phalanx of one or more fingers, and it or they should be applied softly and not pointedly.

The movement starts from the elbow-joint of the manipulator, where there is slight flexion and extension. Between it and the ultimate phalanges of the fingers, the bones of the forearm, wrist, and hands, with their intermediate joints, act, so to speak, as links in a chain, through which a wavelike motion is sent and propagated to the part worked upon.

The movement of the hand is very quick. The joints must not be kept stiff, but just so far extended that elasticity is permitted and not hindered. If this is not attended to, the manipulation becomes hard and pushing. The patient strains his muscles because of the pain and discomfort caused him, and the movement is either productive of bad consequences or has no effect at all.

This manipulation promotes and quickens resorption; it stimulates and strengthens; it diminishes pain by its power to reduce congestion and inflammation; and it increases the secretion of the glands.

It is given for a period varying in length from a few to several minutes, depending upon the disorder and the effect produced.

The illustrations which are appended to the various movements will make it easier to understand how the fingers are applied, and how they work at different portions of the body.

SHAKING OF THE PHARYNX.

There are three different manipulations for the pharynx. and these have already been described by me ("Medical Press and Circular," July 25th, 1888).

1st. The fingers of one hand are placed, with the palmar surface upward, as far back as possible, two on each side of

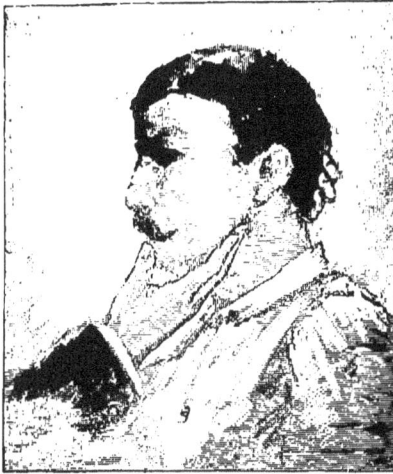

FIG. 20.

the root of the tongue. Then a quick, shaking movement is made in an upward and slightly forward direction (Fig. 20).

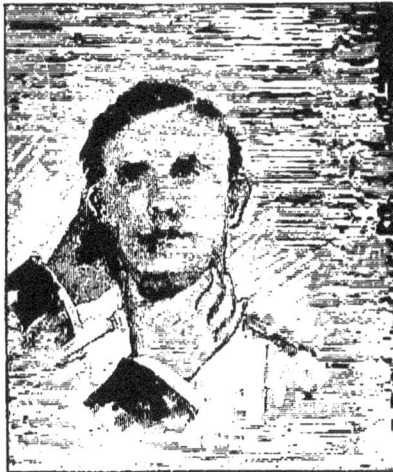

FIG. 21.

If, while giving this shaking, we move our fingers forward, it is evident that the tongue, submaxillary and sublingual glands, will be more especially affected.

2d. The root of the tongue is grasped between the thumb and the fingers, and shaken in a lateral direction (Fig. 21).

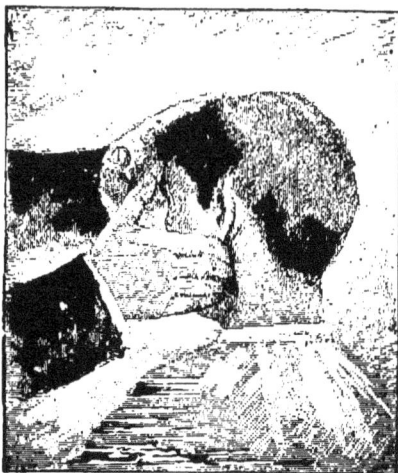

FIG. 22.

3d. The tips of the fingers are placed behind the ascending ramus of the lower jaw (Figs. 22 and 23).

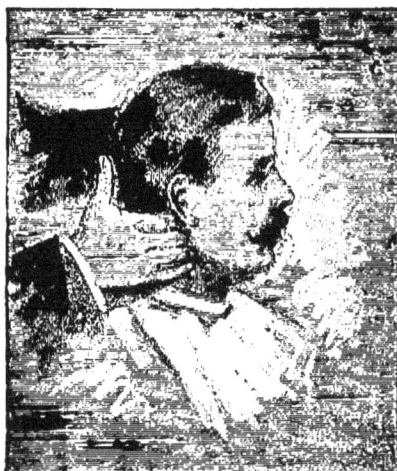

FIG. 23.

Here the movement has the direction inward, forward, and downward. One side may be treated after the other, or both simultaneously, and the operator may either stand in front of or behind the patient. The fingers must be pushed deeply in before the manipulation begins. The greater the distance the motion set up has to pass before it comes to the actual seat of the complaint, the smaller its effect will be.

The head ought to be bent a little forward, in order to relax the cervical fascia and the muscles, which would otherwise prove a considerable hindrance. As a security for this position, the free hand is placed either just above the forehead, or, better still, below the occiput.

The first two movements have in themselves a tendency to bring the head back, and this action is heightened by the patient himself, who instinctively draws away from the working hand, the more so if the complaint from which he is suffering be acute or painful.

When the third manipulation is given with one hand, the head is first turned a little to the opposite side, and then bent toward the one to be treated. This gives a much larger and freer space to work on.

The whole of the pharynx is more or less acted upon by these manipulations, and their effect, if correctly executed, is very rapidly beneficial in nearly all affections of the throat.

Shaking of the Larynx and Upper Part of the Trachea.

The tips of the fingers are placed on one side of the thyroid cartilage, and the thumb on the other (Fig. 24).

The shaking is made sideways. This movement has little effect on the larynx itself, which moves as a whole, but acts more particularly on the part of the trachea below it, as the wave motion passes downward. It is therefore of use in croup and affections of the upper part of the trachea.

If, retaining the same position of the hand, and passing it downward, we make a similar side movement, we act more directly on the trachea itself; and the nearer we approach the sternum the more deeply into the chest is this movement propagated.

Instead of grasping the trachea, we may place two or more fingers on it, in the hollow of the sternum, in the manner shown in Fig. 25. In this manipulation it is of the highest importance that the hand lies close to the throat, in order that the angle formed between the fingers and the trachea may be as small as possible. When the angle is increased, the movement loses its softness; it becomes disagreeable to the patient; the motion produced is, of course, less in the direction of the

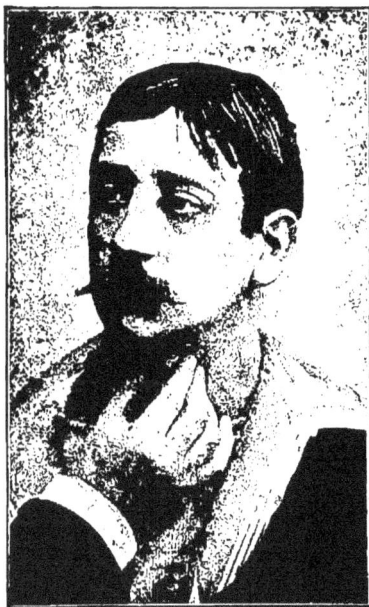

FIG. 24.

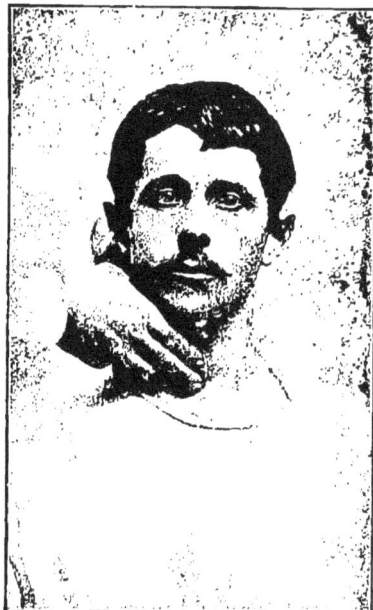

FIG. 25.

trachea, and thus its range of effect becomes more and more limited, until, when the angle is large, the benefit is practically nil.

The patient must sit perfectly upright. The shoulders are to be well thrown back, in order that the respiration may go freely and well.

These shakings, accompanied by tapotement on the chest and between the shoulder-blades, are of very great service in bronchitis and chronic disorders of the lungs.

SHAKINGS OF LOWER PART OF THE THORAX.

The patient stands with the hands folded behind his neck, as in Fig. 26.

The operator places one hand on each side of the lower part of the thorax. With the palms he makes soft and quick

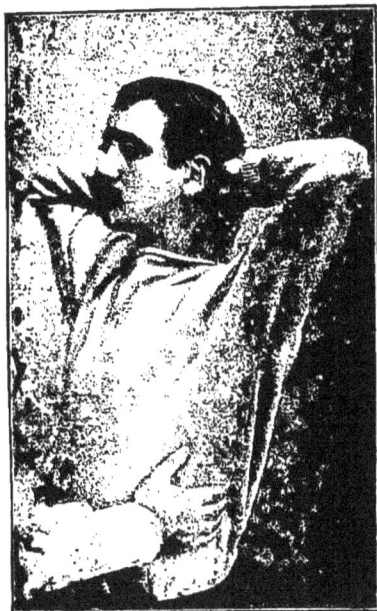

FIG. 26.

compressions, alternating with relaxation. During the latter the hands are not to be lifted from the thorax, but should remain in close contact with it. The patient must breathe deeply. The ribs, being elastic, rebound when the pressure is left off, and the respiration becomes freer and deeper. Besides this, the movement has the influence on pleuritic adhesions at the lower part of the thorax of breaking them down, and the organs in the upper part of the abdominal cavity, below the vault of the diaphragm, are also affected.

This movement is usually given after tapotement of the chest.

Shaking at the Pit of the Stomach.

The patient either stands (Fig. 27), or lies in the recumbent position, as in Fig. 6, in both cases with the hands folded behind his neck. The fingers are placed midway between the ensiform cartilage of the sternum and the navel. We see from the position of the fingers, that they have above them the pyloric part of the stomach and the left lobe of the liver, while

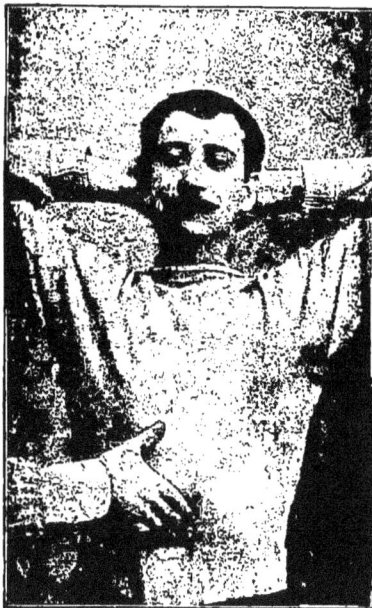

Fig. 27.

just beneath them lies the solar plexus. The movement is made in a backward and slightly upward direction. As the stomach and its continuation, the duodenum, have involuntary muscles in their walls, which are more sensitive to stimulation by reason of their tendency to automatic contraction, and as the solar plexus commands the circulation in the abdomen, we may readily understand that this manipulation must indeed have a great effect. It is therefore used in chronic affections of the stomach and the liver.

Shakings at this spot, when made gently, will relieve

spasms in the diaphragm. For this I have used it with success, both when the cause was reflex, as in hiccough, and in chloroform narcosis.

The stomach and the liver may separately come in for treatment, as we, continuing our shaking, follow the lower border of the thorax to the left or to the right. On our way toward the right there is one place which needs special attention, viz., just under the ninth rib cartilage and the outer

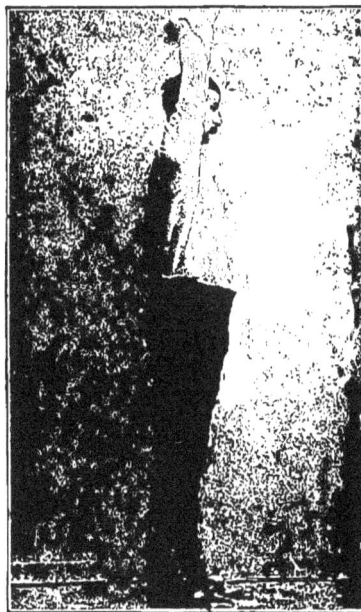

Fig. 28.

border of the rectus abdominalis muscle, where the gall-bladder lies. In patients suffering from impaction of a biliary calculus in the duct, shaking here is sure to be attended with success.

In the recumbent position it is usually given with general pétrissage of the abdomen. When the shaking is administered separately for the liver, the standing side position, as in Fig. 28, is mostly preferred; and in the same attitude, with the left arm raised, the stomach can also be treated.

In derangements of the liver we can in this position work with the left hand between the lower part of the shoulder-

blade of the right side and the spine, where we are certain to
find tender places.

It is always usual to accompany shaking of the liver by
tapotement over the right side of the thorax.

It is evident that when we follow the lower border of the
thorax toward the left, and give the shaking, that the spleen
must also be acted upon. I have seen this mode of treatment
produce marked change for the better in patients suffering
from enlarged spleen, resulting from malaria.

If the hand is spread out over the surface of the abdomen,
and strong shakings made, the whole of the intestine is stimulated to greater activity, the peristaltic movement is increased,
and the secretion from the glands is brisker; and thus they
are indicated in sluggish action of the bowels.

SHAKING OF THE BLADDER.

For the shaking of the bladder we have three positions.
In two—the recumbent and the standing—the manipulation is

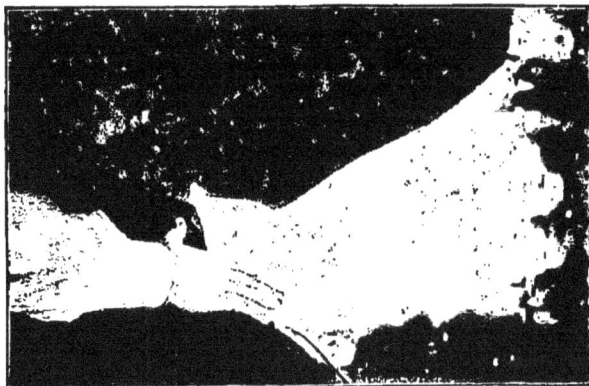

FIG. 29.

given above the pubic arch (Figs. 29 and 30); and in the latter
the patient bends slightly forward, in order to relax the abdominal muscles. In the third he lies in the prone position,
with the legs a little apart, and the toes turned inward in
order to give more room.

When the bladder is acted upon from above, the fingers are
placed about one inch superior to the pubic arch, and the di-

rection of the shaking is from above, downward and backward. In the perineum the fingers are placed just in front of the anal aperture, and the movement passes downward and forward.

By this manipulation we act on the bladder and the prostate, and if we change the direction from below upward in

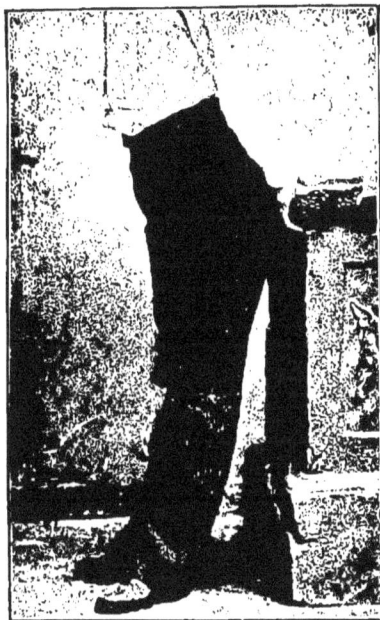

FIG. 30.

the prone position, the lower part of the rectum comes in for treatment.

In the same position, and for females, backward displacements of the uterus are relieved.

This manipulation ought in every case to be followed by the lighter vibration described further on, and by nerve frictions over the sacral, gluteal, and lumbar regions; and should be preceded by tapotement over the same parts.

CHAPTER VIII.

VIBRATIONS.

THE vibrations are, one might say, only fine shaking movements.

The whole or part of the palmar surface of the hand or fingers is used in this kind of manipulation. If we look at the illustration representing vibration of the thorax (Fig. 33), it will be easier to understand its mechanism. Here, as in the shaking, there is flexion and extension at the elbow, but they are much smaller. The movements in the loose wrist-joint are abduction and adduction (*i.e.*, radial and ulnar flexion) of the hand, which lies immovable, so far as the part of the surface of the body on which it rests is concerned. Through the quick succession of the individual movements the vibrations are produced. If flexion and extension are allowed at the wrist, pressure is caused. The injurious influence of this in different localities, say over a weak heart, certainly needs no explanation.

As the vibrations are so often used in order to relieve pain, it is evident how important it is not to work with a stiff hand and wrist. Indeed, the entire advantage of the movement is lost if this be not attended to. On the other hand, when given correctly the vibrations are bound to relieve pain, no matter what the cause of the pain may be.

The straining of the muscles in the operator's arm ought to be so slight as to be scarcely perceptible to any one who has his hand over them.

On no account are the vibrations to be produced by the continued strong contraction of the muscles of the shoulder, arm, and hand. When given thus, the manipulation becomes hard, and the intensity, the acute sensibility that the operator should have of the pressure he is applying, gets lost, while it is impossible to continue the treatment for any length of time, even for a few minutes. The effect over a weak heart is as bad as flexion and extension at the wrist-joint, if not worse. The patient will constantly feel pain, because pressure cannot be avoided, and maybe he will faint.

I will give a few instances in which one can perceive the difference between a movement produced by strong contraction of the muscles of the arm—which of course carries with it an immovable wrist and hand—and the way in which I have described it:

1. Place the hand on the thigh. In the first kind of manipulation a harder grip of the muscles is necessary, the muscular mass moves as a whole, there are no vibrations just under the place of application of the hand, the range of the movement produced is much smaller; while in the second, the hand lies loosely on the surface, the vibrations pass into and are felt in the underlying muscles, and are widely propagated.

2. You may give vibrations to the anterior surface of the thorax, and feel them in the other hand placed on the back of the patient, while with the stiff arm and hand you feel nothing at all.

3. Place a glass of water in the middle of a fairly large table. Make the vibrations, and if the water moves as a whole from side to side they are made wrongly, but if the surface of the water quickens in the centre only they are made correctly.

This may give an idea of how delicate the movements really are, and how it is possible to use them in disorders where shakings and the ordinary massage manipulations are entirely out of question.

The vibrations have a much greater effect than the shakings in the production of resorption, and especially in diminishing pain, both of which can be seen in congestions and acute and chronic inflammatory conditions.

VIBRATIONS OF THE EYES.

There are two kinds:

1. The patient closes the eyes, and the operator, standing behind him, lays two of the fingers on each eye, and commences the vibrations (Fig. 31). He has to take care that the eyelids do not move up and down, but are kept steady on the eyeball, so that the vibrations pass through them.

2. We may place the distal phalanx of the thumb on the

outer side of one eye, and the same phalanx of the fore and long fingers on the outer side of the other eye (as seen in Fig.

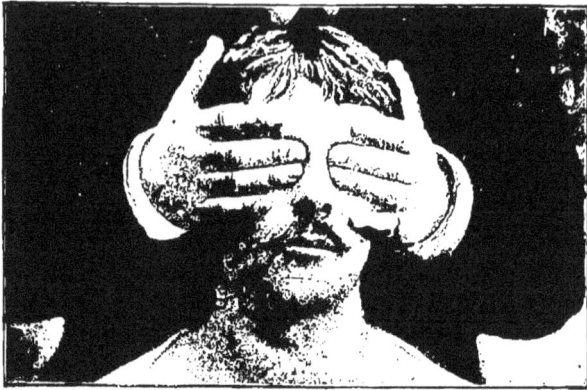

FIG. 31.

32), and make the vibrations. They ought to be felt deeply through the eyeballs.

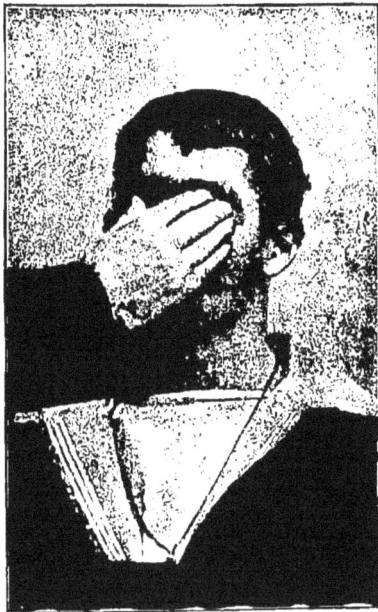

FIG. 32.

The first movement, which does not penetrate so deep, affects the superficial parts, while by the latter the deeper parts are more acted upon. They should always be accompanied by frictions and vibrations over all the sensory nerves round the eye, and also by frictions on the eyeball itself, as will be described later on.

I have found these movements to be of great benefit in affections of the cornea and conjunctiva, not only in relieving the inflammation, pain, and photophobia, but also in accelerating the healing process.

VIBRATIONS OF THE THROAT.

When vibrations are given for ailments of the throat, the fingers are placed in the same position as for shakings; and the former are here always substituted for the latter at the beginning of acute inflammation.

As there are many glands in this region, I may at this point state that whenever enlarged glands are treated by the manual method, these vibrations should be used, and they will not be had recourse to in vain.

VIBRATIONS OF THE LARYNX.

For the larynx the application of the fingers is the same as shown in Fig. 24, and it is evident that the vibrations have a direct effect on the larynx itself, while the shakings tend to pass over it.

VIBRATIONS ON THE THORAX.

The position of the patient should be either lying down straight on his back, with the hands clasped behind the neck, or standing up, as in Fig. 33.

The place of application of the hand in giving vibrations for the thorax, varies with the nature of the disorder we are treating. The whole hand is here used. It lies loose and free, without pressure, on the thoracic wall. The vibrations pass through the thoracic wall to the lungs, which they stimulate and strengthen. They produce free expectoration, followed by less irritation, promote rest and a feeling of ease, and, when administered in conjunction with nerve frictions between the shoulder-blades, etc., also reduce congestive and

inflammatory conditions. The vibrations on the thorax are
given for all diseases of the lungs, and they must be continued
for some minutes.

It may be interesting in this connection to mention a case
that recently came under my care. Last January, a young
gentleman, twenty-two years old, consulted me on the subject
of a constant dry and hacking cough with which he was
troubled. In February, 1888, during a stay in India, he had

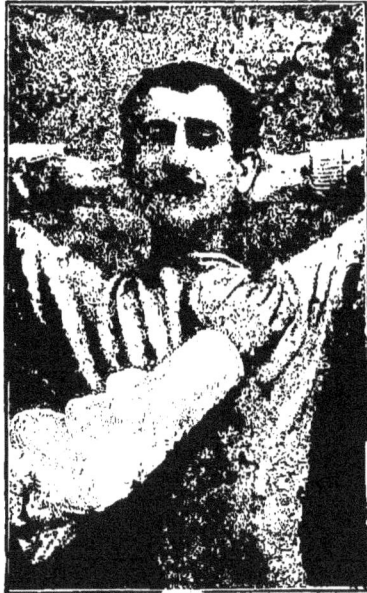

FIG. 33.

contracted a cold, and the cough had remained with him since,
gradually increasing in severity. The patient had previously
been in South Africa, where he had gone through an acute
attack of fever. In the spring of 1889 he returned to Africa,
where he soon fell a victim to dysentery, and was dangerously
ill for six weeks. It was not considered possible for him to
continue out there, so he returned home in the autumn. The
patient did not rally properly, but remained very thin and
pale; the cough grew more intense, and greatly troubled him
at night. He had attacks of dysentery at least once a week.
In company with the increase of the cough came breathless-

ness on walking quickly or going up-stairs, a feeling of lassi-
tude, and profuse sweating—the patient, to use his own expression, being bathed in perspiration. Deep inspiration gave
pain at the tip of both the lungs, more so on the right side;
same on coughing. Respiration was short and quick—even
up to thirty-eight in the minute. Slight dulness at both the
apices — more marked on the right side. Appetite not
good.

The lung symptoms were treated with vibrations and tapotement of the thorax, movements causing deep respiration,
nerve frictions, and tapotement between the shoulder-blades,
especially at the upper part, where the patient was very sensitive; the dysentery with vibrations and general pétrissage
of the abdomen. In addition, the patient received some general treatment including nerve frictions.

The cough gradually passed away; the sweating during
the night ceased; the respiration grew deep and free—sixteen
to eighteen a minute; no breathlessness; the appetite was
good. During the time he was under treatment the patient
had no attack of dysentery. He has enjoyed excellent health
ever since.

The treatment lasted a fortnight.

VIBRATIONS OVER THE HEART.

If we are to give vibrations over the heart, they must be
given very carefully, the hand being placed lightly over the
apex. Just as their effect is good when properly executed, so
the result is mischievous when they are unskilfully performed.
A weak heart has already more than enough work to do, and
if a heavy hand is added, rendered still heavier by a stiff wrist,
together with flexion and extension at the same place, it is no
wonder the patient feels anything but ease, and frequently
pain, and sometimes even faints.

According to the condition of the patient, he may lie or
stand—the arms may be up or down, and the hands fixed behind the neck (Fig. 33)—but the chest must always be well
thrown out.

The effect of the vibrations is a stronger, quieter, and better beat. This is well seen in a fainting fit when the heart
stops or begins to flag, and also in the opposite condition, viz.,

4

palpitation. During the former, the beat soon comes back or grows stronger; while in the latter steadiness in its action returns.

In fainting from shock, the simplest method of reviving the patient is to compress the internal jugular veins.

Vibrations of the Abdomen, or Part of it.

For vibrations of the abdomen in general, the position of the patient and the position of the hand are precisely the same as in pétrissage. For special situations, part of the palm and fingers, or the back of the fingers of the lightly-closed hand, are used.

These vibrations are valuable in relieving pain and stopping diarrhœa, whatever the cause of these may be; but they should never be given in cases of constipation, for they tend to produce this condition.

In connection with the action of vibrations of the abdomen on diarrhœa, I may mention the case of a gentleman, about fifty-seven years old, who suffered from this complaint. For five or six weeks he had felt pain and discomfort in the abdomen generally. During day and night he had frequent calls to stool, and the motions were constantly mingled with blood. After two treatments his bowels acted perfectly normal, and the pains had of course disappeared.

A friend of mine, a young Swedish officer, whom I met while at Stockholm last autumn, had suffered intensely from diarrhœa for some weeks before he mentioned the fact to me. He was growing seriously pale and thin. I treated him for the first time one evening before he went to bed. The night that followed that treatment was the first during which he had complete rest for over a fortnight; while previously he had been obliged to rise several times every night. I continued the treatment for a few days; and during the four or five weeks I afterward stayed in Stockholm he had no relapse.

As regards pain, I have relieved it both in colic, in acute general peritonitis, and perityphlitis. The effect of vibrations in causing constipation is of marked advantage in cases of this kind, where action of the bowels is contra-indicated.

For the bladder, it is better to use the back of the flexed fingers, and the hand should be well down in the pelvis.

At the pit of the stomach we have recourse to vibrations in painful gastric conditions, such as ulcer, acute catarrh, and nervous dyspepsia. They probably produce their effect through the solar plexus of the sympathetic.

When we use them for pain at the menstrual period, p.-p. hemorrhage, metritis, endometritis, etc., the uterus must be grasped between the fingers and the thumb, and quick and light frictions made at the same time as the vibrations. This mode of treatment dispenses with the internal manipulation in the above-named disorders.

In vibrations for affections of the anus, such as hemorrhoids and prolapsus, the last phalanx of one or more fingers is used. In prolapsus ani, the tips of the fingers are placed round the protruding mass before the vibrations begin.

In treatment of piles it is not sufficient to apply local treatment; but shaking of the liver, pétrissage of the abdomen, etc., must also be resorted to.

VIBRATIONS OVER ULCERS.

It is necessary to cover the ulcer with a piece of linen or lint moistened with some antiseptic solution, and over this again some gutta-percha, in order to prevent the heat of the hand from passing to the ulcer. The palm of the hand is afterward applied, and the vibrations made. These have to be combined with pétrissage round the ulcer, in order that the parts surrounding it may be kept healthy, and stimulated to greater activity.

VIBRATIONS FOR FURENCLES AND ABSCESSES.

The tips of the fingers and thumb are placed at the periphery of the affected tissues, and during vibrations are approximated to each other, passing gradually toward the middle. The effect of this is to drive the degenerated blood serum to the centre, and pointing takes place quicker. When the abscess has been opened, this manipulation removes the pus from the abscess cavity more completely and painlessly than by the ordinary method of pressure.

CHAPTER IX.

IN the "Medical Press and Circular" of July 25th, 1888, I have already spoken about the different ways of causing nerve vibrations, and perhaps I may be allowed to quote what I then said: "The manipulator causes the nerve to vibrate either by frictions made transversely over it, in a manner similar to that in which a harp-player passes his fingers over the strings of his harp; or he makes vibrations over the nerve. When the latter method is adopted, he either follows its course with the tips of his fingers in a centripetal direction, or he keeps them fixed, and vibrates upon such parts of it as are more painful.

"The different methods of procedure (frictions or vibrations) depend upon the position and surroundings of the nerve. Nervus medianus is very suitable for demonstration of the first. The arm is abducted until it reaches the horizontal position. The nerve coming out of the axilla can be easily felt as a thick cord lying to the outside of the bronchial artery. When the tips of the fingers are quickly drawn over it transversely in the manner indicated above, a feeling is produced similar to that felt on electric stimulation. Nervus supraorbitalis, which lies on the bone, is a good instance where the second kind of procedure may be employed.

"It is essential that the tissues which lie between the fingers and the nerve should move with the former as one; otherwise the friction does not reach its destination, and the manipulation becomes useless.

"According to my own experience, the effects of this mechanical method are, so far as I can judge—

"1. *Raising of the nervous energy.*

"2. *Diminution of pain* (as seen in facial neuralgia, sciatica, migraine, and similar disorders).

"3. *Contraction of the smaller blood-vessels.* (Heaviness

of the head is quickly relieved by stimulation of the sensory nerves of the scalp. Frictions over the sensory branches of the cervical and brachial plexuses in the neck produce in nearly every person a chilly feeling passing down over the body, often accompanied by cutis anserina.)

"4. *Stimulation of the muscles to contraction.* (In several persons in a weak condition, and some whose nervous system was highly irritable, I have seen this well marked; frictions over the N. musculo-spiralis being followed by corresponding flexion and extension of the wrist, and also of the fingers.)"

I may mention that in a lady patient, whom I have seen during the last weeks of my stay at Pola, and who suffered from spastic (reflex) paraplegia, whose inferior extremities had remained stiffly extended for nearly five years, after a difficult child-bed, contraction of the muscles and flexion of the legs instantly followed stimulation of the nerves of the leg and those under the foot. They returned to their extended position when the stimulation ceased; but, after treatment for a few times, the feet could be separated for a distance of about 20 cm., and the stiffness of the knee and ankle was not so absolute as before. I can add—

"5. *Increased secretion of the glands.* (Frictions over the facial nerve, or in the situation where the submaxillary ganglion lies, are instantly followed by increase of the secretion of saliva.)

"6. *Diminished excretion from the skin.* I have often noticed while treating patients with frictions over the cervical nerves that the perspiration which at first has been perceptible all over the body has quickly disappeared under the influence of these movements, and that free perspiration in the palms of the hands has passed away on frictions being applied to the median nerve.

"7. *Decrease of temperature.* This is well marked in fevers and feverish conditions.

"As regards pressure on the nerves, I have found it very useful in many cases of migraine and neuralgia. The pressure was kept up for a period varying from a few to several minutes at the time, and after a slight interval renewed, the whole lasting from five to twenty minutes."

My brother, Mr. Henrik Kellgren, has, during the last twenty years, worked out and greatly developed this system

of direct mechanical stimulation of the nerves. Ling and his
pupils had already an idea of this method, as is shown by the
writings of Georgii (" Traitement des maladies par le mouve-
ment," Paris, 1847).

They had noticed the effect of frictions applied from the
front backward in the line of the longitudinal sinus, and also
of the lateral one. They found that these frictions produced
not only a contraction of the skin on the cranium, but also a

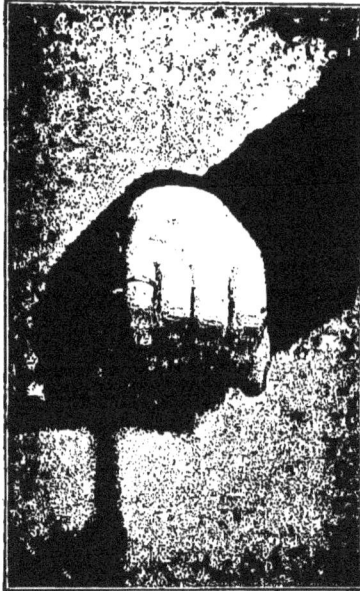

FIG. 34.

shivering feeling down the back, and they used them with
success in several cases of fulness of blood in the head and
congestion of the brain.

The fingers and the thumb are kept slightly bent, so that
the back of the nails come in contact with the scalp, and with
light vibrations they are passed backward (Fig. 34). When
they arrive at the occipital protuberance, the fingers follow
the direction of one of the lateral sinuses, the thumb that of
the other.

That the effect of these vibrations should be considerable,
we can deduce from the feeling they produce; as also from

the fact that all the sensory nerves of the scalp pass up to the vertex, and are thus acted upon.

These frictions ought never to be omitted in a general treatment of the head. With them we must give movements which draw the blood away from the head or toward it, according to the requirements of the case.

Ling and his pupils also tried frictions over the phrenic and great sciatic nerves. The former they manipulated, in order to relieve spasm of the diaphragm. This is easier, and with greater certainty allayed by light shakings in the pit of the stomach, as was well seen in a patient at the Marine Hospital at Pola, who during chloroform narcosis was seized with this spasm. The shakings had the direction from below upward and backward.

Whenever a sensory nerve is stimulated by electricity, it causes contraction of the blood-vessels. Since these frictions over the median and several other nerves give exactly the same feeling as that from an electrical shock, and as the chilly sensation passing over the body, accompanied with cutis anserina, must be caused by contraction of the smaller blood-vessels of the skin, these frictions, with their consequent vibrations, must produce the same effect as the electrical stimulation does. I have taken this as the guiding idea for the use of this form of nerve stimulation, and the results certainly seem to justify the belief.

We must take care, however, before this mechanical stimulation is applied, either to feel the nerve or be perfectly certain as to its topographical situation, and to be well down on it when it lies deeply, as, for instance, in the case of the great sciatic in the gluteal region.

When we have to do with a muscular or mixed nerve, and our intention is merely to stimulate it in an ordinary way, we give frictions, and may pass up and down its course; but when pain is present, or the nerve purely sensory, vibrations alone, or followed by constant pressure, are to be preferred. The vibrations are then administered as previously described. We ought also to remember, that we have often several nerves coming from the same plexus, and that although only one branch of a nerve may seem to give pain, the other nerves or branches send their stimulation to the same centre, and thus act reflexly on the affected nerve or branch.

There is no doubt but that in these nerve vibrations, combined with other passive and active movements, a powerful weapon has been given us against the progress of most of the nervous diseases. I have seen several cases of paralysis, locomotor ataxia, spastic paralysis, infantine paralysis, etc., which have been greatly relieved. The result of the manual method in these and other nervous diseases would be still more successful if the patients had recourse to the treatment sooner. At present it is used as the last plank after everything else has failed. Not only have we then to contend with the diseases in their very advanced stages, but also with the sunken courage and lost energy of the patient, which react so unfavorably on his general health.

I may now proceed to give some directions as to the best and easiest places to find the different nerves.

NERVES OF THE HEAD AND NECK.

Nervus Occipitalis Major, Nervus Occipitalis Minor, and Nervus Auricularis Major.

These are all branches of the second pair of cervical nerves, the latter also having a root from the third pair. We find them best a little below the lower half of the mastoid process (Fig. 35). Frictions there cause a feeling of coldness to run down over the body; and if they are made strongly, pain is felt, not only at the points of application of the fingers, but also inside the head, as far forward as the frontal region, and up on the vertex.

Treatment of these nerves relieves headache and congestion of the brain, and its effect is extremely good in hemicrania, sleeplessness, etc. In migraine, the above-mentioned feeling of pain is most beautifully demonstrated. I have, with treatment of these nerves, also cured severe headaches in fevers. During my stay at Pola there was a slight epidemic of cerebro-spinal meningitis. A naval officer was brought to the hospital, suffering from this disease. He had had for four days and nights most severe headache and fever. Antipyrine, subcutaneous injections of morphia, and other remedies, had been tried, but the headache did not diminish, nor did he obtain sleep. I was asked to try to relieve him. I gave him frictions over these nerves, alternating with constant pressure, vibrations on the vertex in the line of the longitudinal sinus, as described before, together with some other passive movements which lead the blood from the head, and finished up with general pétrissage of the abdomen. After the first treatment in the morning, the headache disappeared, and the patient slept for some hours. I treated him again in the afternoon and evening. As the latter approached, he had oc-

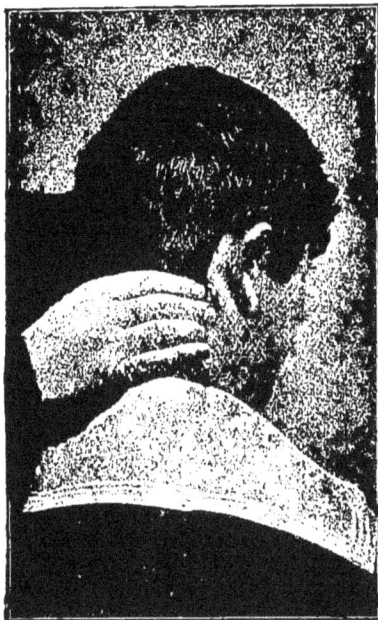

Fig. 35.

casionally slight headache, but it soon passed away. After the last treatment he felt free in his head. During the night he slept well, and the following morning had no headache. The headache did not reappear.

At first, vibrations should be made for several minutes, and then an immovable constant pressure kept up with the fingers. The patient feels at first severe pain in the head, but this either passes entirely away during the manipulation, or disappears very shortly after the cessation of treatment. When there is congestion of the brain and fulness of blood, all the nerves of the scalp should be treated.

NERVUS SUPRAORBITALIS.

This nerve is best found at the supraorbital notch or foramen. If there is a notch, the nerve is easy to find; but when
it passes through a foramen it is best reached by placing the
tip of the fore or long finger in the orbit, and feeling it as it
lies against the roof just before it goes into the foramen. In
these two situations, it is better to make frictions over it with

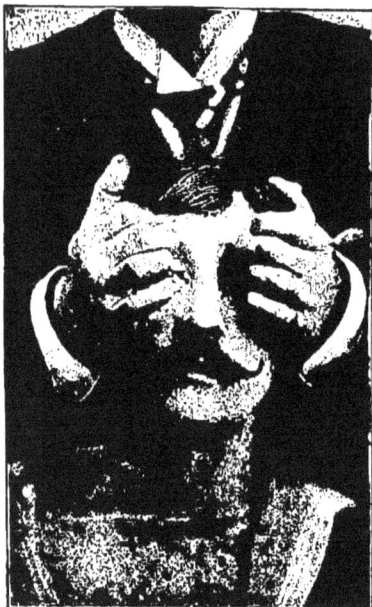

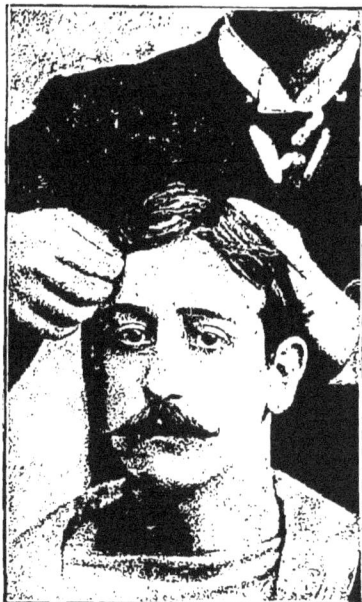

FIG. 36.   FIG. 37.

the back part of the nail, taking care not to apply the edge.
(Note the strong bending of the last phalanx in Fig. 36.)

On the forehead we first trace the nerve from the notch
upward under light frictions, and we find it lying like a thin
cord, curving somewhat outward toward the temples. Having delineated its course, the vibrations are begun, and made
time after time in the centripetal direction (Fig. 37).

Fig. 38 shows how the thumb is applied to the forefinger
when we work with the back of its nail, viz., not at the very
tip, but nearer the last phalangeal joint. This imparts greater
softness to the manipulation.

For neuralgia in this nerve, it is often enough to treat it alone; but if this is not successful, I give vibrations over the other branches from the same nerve stem.

NERVUS SUPRATROCHLEARIS AND NERVUS NASALIS.

The supratrochlear nerve comes out at the inner part of the orbit, and it runs nearly vertically upward.

The nasal nerve is found to emerge on the side of the nose at the nasal bone with the cartilage.

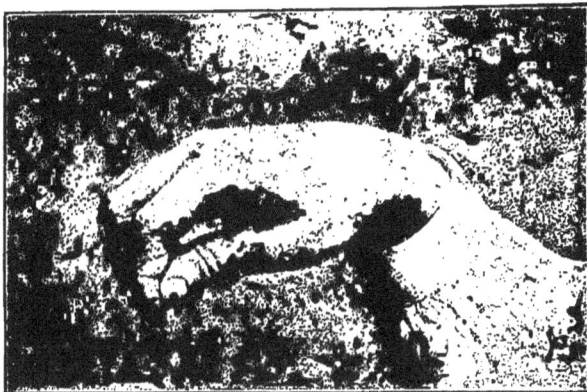

FIG. 38.

Vibrations over these two nerves are very beneficial in catarrh of the nose, cold in the head, and its accompaniment, frontal headache.

A sensory twig, probably from the lachrymal nerve, turns round the edge of the orbit at its outer side, just opposite the outer canthus. Light frictions or vibrations there cause, even in sound persons, considerable irritation, while on those who have any affection of the eye the pain is very pronounced.

NERVUS MAXILLARIS SUPERIOR AND NERVUS MENTALIS.

If we pass down in a straight line from the supraorbital notch, we have no difficulty in finding these nerves, where they come out of their respective foramina. I have cured neuralgic toothache at once; and even in cases where the tooth has been

diseased, the pain often subsided when vibrations were applied
over the nerves for a few minutes. I have also by the same
treatment stopped the aching in the teeth and jaws following
on strong mercurial inunction.

NERVUS FACIALIS.

Frictions can most easily be applied to the facial nerve
where it comes forward over the ascending ramus of the in-

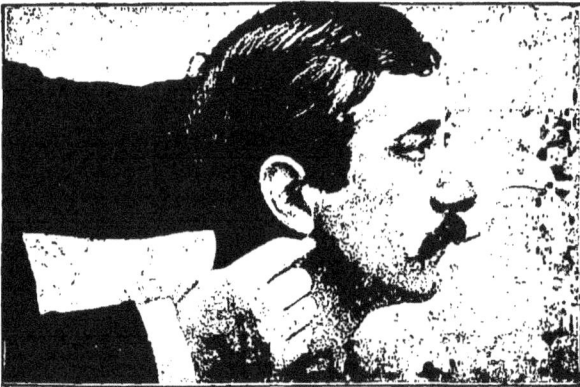

FIG. 39.

ferior maxillary bone.   They are made from above downward
(Fig. 39).

The first effect, on friction being applied, is a peculiar
sparkling sensation, not only over the side of the face, but also
in the pharynx, and very frequently, too, in the ear.

This nerve, of course, should be stimulated in cases of facial
paralysis.

While working under my brother, I had occasion to see two
cases of complete recovery.   One of the patients was a little
boy, five years old, the other a girl of fourteen.

In all disorders of the throat, this nerve comes in for treatment, not only because of its connection with the pharynx, but
also in order to produce increased flow of saliva from the
parotid gland.

Nervus Lingualis.

In order to find the lingual nerve, we must bend the head a little to that side on which the nerve which is to be subjected to treatment is situated, and the friction is made from within outward. This also increases the secretion of saliva from the submaxillary glands.

If the patient sits with his head erect, and if we make a friction from behind forward between the submaxillary gland and the bone, a sparkling sensation indicates that the submaxillary ganglion has been touched.

Nerve Frictions and Vibrations on the Eyeball itself.

The patient is told to look downward, and then to close the eyes. The tip of the forefinger is placed on the upper part of

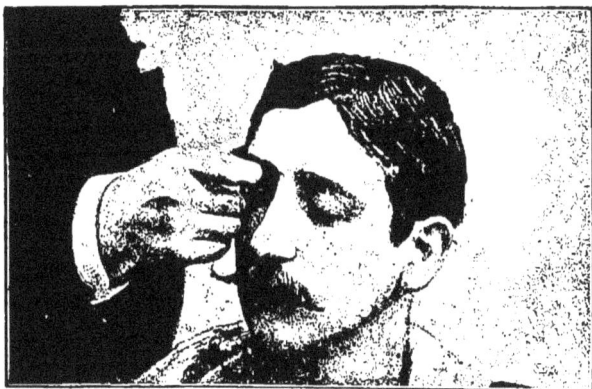

Fig 40.

the eye, just to the inner side of the vertical diameter of the eyeball (Fig. 40).

Light frictions here cause a strong sensation, which is felt not only in the eye itself, but may even be experienced inside the skull at its anterior part.

At other places on the eye, the feeling is not so well marked. The patient has more the sensation of having sand in the eye.

These nerves are to be stimulated in affections of the eye, and also in migraine and ordinary headache. In a patient

who had lost a great deal of blood, and, following on this, suffered from a very severe headache, I had recourse to these
vibrations on both eyes simultaneously, since all other treatment seemed of no avail. I was obliged to give the frictions
for about fifteen minutes before the headache ceased entirely.

Nervus Laryngeus Superior.

This nerve is easily reached where it lies below the great
cornua of the hyoid bone, and before it pierces the thyro-hyoid

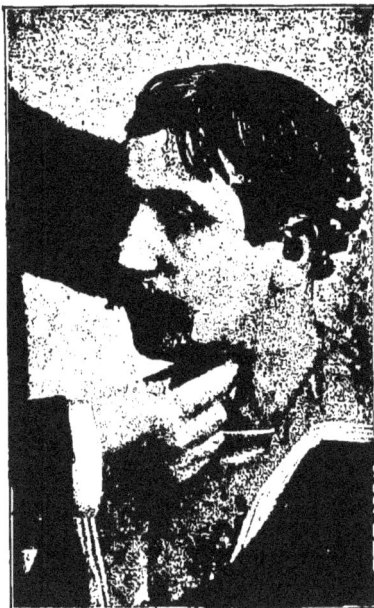

Fig. 41.

membrane. The finger tip is placed at the posterior end of
the upper border of the thyroid cartilage, and quickly drawn
forward (Fig. 41).

Pain is felt at the place of application, in the larynx, often
in the ear and pharynx, and up in the head. Indeed, when I
practise this treatment on myself, and continue it for a few
seconds, I feel either pain or prickling in these places; and in
the brain I have a sensation as if a strong band were bound
round it.

These nerves must be stimulated in affections of the larynx.

Nervus Laryngeus Inferior.

The head should be bent toward the side on which lies the nerve to be stimulated, and slightly forward. The finger is passed down beside the trachea to the inner side of the lower part of the sterno-mastoid muscle, and the friction is made toward the windpipe. Administered to healthy persons, it generally causes cough.

Nervus Vagus.

The vagus nerve lies in the sheath between the carotid artery and the internal jugular vein. We must have the head flexed a little forward, and feel for the pulsating artery. The finger is placed just outside it, carefully pressed downward, and afterward quick and sharp frictions are made transversely. In a patient with bronchitis or allied affection, this nearly always produces cough, and it should be given in combination with shaking of the trachea. Its effect on the heart is utilized when the action of the latter is too strong; and this effect must be taken into consideration in treating patients with weak hearts, or fainting may ensue. In derangements of the stomach and liver, frictions over this nerve often produce vomiting.

First Cervical Sympathetic Ganglion.

We stand behind the patient, whose head is at first slightly bent backward. The finger is then passed high up inside the angle of the lower jaw. We next flex the head forward, and as the cervical fascia relaxes, we pass the finger upward and backward until we reach the front of the vertebral column. The finger is now passed quickly from side to side, when pain is produced, varying in sharpness and extent of distribution according to the force with which the friction is given. The pain may be felt on the whole side of the head and pharynx. I have several times had patients under my hands, who, from frictions not over strong, have had a feeling of fainting. If the wideness of the distributing and connecting branches of the nerve are taken into consideration, these results may to some extent be accounted for.

CERVICAL NERVES.

Here, also, just as is shown in the illustration of nerve frictions over the second cervical pair (Fig. 35), we use the tips of the fingers on one side, and the last phalanx of the thumb on the other. We place them on the edges of the trapezius muscle. A sharp and quick friction is made at the same time as the tips of the fingers are approximated to that of the thumb. I have often seen, or rather felt, that new beginners have the habit of using equal pressure, or they push the fingers into the neck. On no account should this be done. The primary cause of the error, as in so many other cases of faulty manipulation, lies in the stiffness in the fingers and hands. This only gives pain, which is very unnecessary, instead of producing the symptom of correct application—*i.e.*, a cold feeling running down over the body.

As we pass down the neck, the distance between the points of application of the tips of the fingers and the thumb is somewhat increased; otherwise the frictions fall inside the places where the sensory nerves lie freer, and no effect at all is produced.

We must take advantage of these nerve frictions in fevers. It is then necessary to continue them for several minutes, the duration, of course, being dependent on the severity of the case.

For my own part, I always direct my attention specially to the places where the second pair of cervical nerves emerge.

NERVES OF THE TRUNK.

LATERAL AND ANTERIOR CUTANEOUS BRANCHES OF THE INTERCOSTAL NERVES.

If we make frictions somewhat obliquely from above downward over each intercostal space, a little anterior to a longitudinal line drawn midway between the anterior and posterior folds of the axilla, we shall find the lateral cutaneous branches of the intercostal nerves.

The anterior cutaneous branches of the intercostal nerves, from the second, third, and fourth, are especially large, and supply many branches to the mammary gland.

These anterior intercostal cutaneous branches are at once found where they come out in the intercostal spaces near the sternum.

Stimulation of these nerves and of the descending cervicals, passing down over the clavicle, is of importance, because they not only supply the skin over the chest, but also the mammary gland; and hence there are often shooting pains toward the neck and arms in inflammatory and other diseased conditions of the gland.

For the summer, 1885, I had charge of my brother's institution in London. A lady, about forty years of age, residing at Kensington, came for the treatment, having a hard lump at the upper and outer part of the left mamma. The skin was somewhat retracted, and could not be separated from the tumor.

This had been forming for some months, and was now an inch and a half in diameter. The patient complained of severe pain, which, when at its height, also passed down the left arm, and prevented her from sleeping.

The movements I prescribed were: Vibrations over the above-named nerves to be continued for five minutes; vibrations on the tumor itself for twenty minutes or more, until the pain was relieved; and a general treatment of active movements.

The patient was treated twice a day, having the special movements only in the evening. At the end of nine months she very seldom felt any pain. The tumor had gone, and only some fibrous strings could be felt at the original site of the swelling.

DORSAL SENSORY NERVES.

When we make frictions over the dorsal sensory nerves, the patient usually lies in the prone position, as for tapotement of the back; in fact, we seldom give the latter alone, but usually precede it with the former method of treatment. The hands of the operator are held somewhat differently, depending on the place where they are applied. Between the shoulders, the back of the forefinger nail, steadied by the thumb, as seen in Fig. 38, is used, because otherwise it is very difficult in this position to give a good friction.

Below and above this point, the palmar surface of the last

5

phalanx is worked with. The direction of the friction is obliquely from below, upward or outward, or the reverse—as,
for instance, if the patient lies on his back, and has the frictions
after general pétrissage of the abdomen. For the general
treatment of these nerves both hands are used at the same
time (one on each side), and we generally pass up and down
the back three or four times, pausing here and there over
places that may be painful, and consequently need more
special manipulation.

One ought not to pass carelessly up and down the back, or
discard frictions in this region without full trial. It must be
remembered that every pair of sensory nerves, springing as
they do from the posterior primary divisions of the spinal
nerves, may be regarded as being each in connection with its
own segment of the spinal cord, while we must also bear in
mind the intimate relations between the spinal nerves and the
sympathetic ganglia. Indeed, it is found that in patients with
heart disease or acute affections of the lungs, the region between the shoulders is very sensitive, and the effect of continued frictions extremely beneficial. I do not wish to be
considered as saying too much before others have had the
same experience, but I have, and my brother before me,
treated cases of pneumonia with nerve frictions between the
shoulders and vibrations on the thorax for the lungs, nerve
frictions in the neck and over the dorsal sensory nerves for the
fever and headache, and pétrissage of the abdomen for the
circulation generally, without help of medicine, and have
always succeeded. Any one who has some little knowledge
of the treatment, may easily obtain confirmation of the fact
that the sensory nerves on the side corresponding to the
diseased lung respond very painfully indeed, while on the
other side frictions give very little pain.

In disorders of the liver, we find tender places corresponding to the lower angle of the scapula on the right side. I may
give an instance of the effect of stimulation of the nerves in
this situation. Doct. Med. Eugen. Gruber, surgeon in the
Imperial Austrian Navy, had a patient who suffered from
biliary calculus. The patient had had several attacks, during
which the pain had been reduced by injections of morphia.
Some little time ago these attacks returned; the patient was
again obliged, as heretofore, to take to her bed, and suffered

very much. Dr. Gruber prescribed, as usual, subcutaneous injections. The pain was not relieved, although two injections were administered. Then he remembered what I had shown, and tried nerve frictions. In the back, as described, he easily found some very tender places. He made frictions over them. They at once produced a strong fit of vomiting, the pain was relieved, and the patient was better.

In diseases of the kidney we have to turn our attention to the lower dorsal nerves. When the generative organs, the bladder, and the rectum are affected, we also find tender places in the lumbar and sacral regions. There are two places in the lumbar region which respond very readily to frictions, viz., just below the twelfth rib, at the angle formed by it and the deeper muscles of the back, and at the base of the spine, where an angle is formed by the same muscles and the crest of the os ilium.

A lady, 27 years old, married, no children, had from the very first suffered agonizing pain at each menstrual period. The pain set in two or three days before the catamenial flow began, and continued throughout the whole period, leaving her completely exhausted for several days. During the attack she was confined to her bed, and could often not lie down, but was obliged to sit up, and she was able to obtain very little sleep. The abdomen—especially its lower part—was painful to the touch. The patient had become anæmic, weak, and nervous.

The special treatment applied was nerve frictions at the upper and lower parts of the lumbar regions and over the sacrum, and vibrations on the lower parts of the abdomen. In addition, some general movements were given.

The treatment extended over three menstrual periods, beginning shortly before one, and finishing a few days after the third.

Her condition had already during the first improved to such an extent that she could come to see me every day. During the second period she had only one attack of pain, and at the third she suffered no pain whatever. The general condition had greatly improved.

If we look at the anatomical arrangement of the nerves, it gives a possible reason for these conditions. The sympathetic ganglia in the neck have communicating branches with all the cervical spinal nerves, and each ganglion gives a nerve to the cardiac plexus. In the dorsal region the sympathetic ganglia all communicate with the corresponding spinal nerves, and the upper five ganglia send branches to the thoracic viscera, through the medium of the cardiac and pulmonary plexuses; while from the sixth to the tenth dorsal ganglia, branches unite to form the great splanchnic, which passes to the semilunar ganglia of the solar plexus. The tenth and eleventh ganglia give origin to the small splanchnic, which joins the solar and renal plexuses; and from the twelfth ganglia arises the smallest splanchnic, which enters the renal plexus.

The same intimate connections also exist between the sympathetic and the lumbar and sacral spinal nerves.

Reflexly, we ought then to be able to react on the organs supplied from the different sympathetic plexuses, as well as to relieve pain in the corresponding sensory nerves.

Over the sacrum the same position of the hand is used as between the shoulders; or the hand is lightly closed, and we work with the knuckles. The nerves here should always be stimulated after the shaking and vibration movements in derangements of the pelvic organs.

We should not forget, in general nerve treatment of the back, to follow the crest of the os ilium, and to give frictions where the topographical anatomy teaches us that the sensory branches of the last dorsal nerve, ilio-hypogastric nerve, and upper lumbar nerves pass downward. When the frictions are correctly made, *i.e.*, a little obliquely, these nerves respond readily.

NERVES OF THE LOWER EXTREMITY.

Nervus Ischiadicus Major.

This is far the most important nerve in the lower extremity. It emerges, as we know, through the great sacro-sciatic foramen beneath the gluteus maximus, and lying nearly midway between the great trochanter of the femur and the tuberosity of the ischium, it passes straight down the back of the thigh to the popliteal space.

The patient is placed in the prone position, as shown in Fig. 5, and the foot of the leg to be treated is crossed over the other. We have here a position in which we can manipulate all the nerves on the back of the limb most readily, because all the muscles from those of the gluteal region down to the calf are more or less relaxed.

If we wish only to stimulate the nerve in a general treatment, and when there is no particular pain, then a few quick frictions should be made over the nerve, while we follow its course upward and downward. I must repeat here, what I have said before, that care must be taken not to make the friction before one is well down upon the nerve, or feels it, as in the popliteal space. On the other hand, if we have to do with a patient who suffers from such a complaint as sciatica, it is better to put the last phalanx of the thumb over the nerve where it emerges from the pelvis, and to make vibrations there. In recent cases of sciatica I have treated, I proceeded in this way, and the consequences for the better were really remarkable. In order to take the vibrations on their own merit, I gave nothing else at the beginning. Not only did the pain diminish and nearly disappear after my first treatment, but the improvement was sustained; and where the patients had been racked with pain day and night, they obtained rest and could sleep.

In the popliteal space, at its upper part, the nerve divides into the internal and external popliteal nerves.

The internal, passing as it does right through the popliteal space, is easily felt, and there is little or no difficulty in applying frictions to it. When it passes down into the calf as posterior tibial, and is covered by the large muscles of that region, we must take care that these move with our fingers. Behind the internal malleolus, it lies with the artery quite superficially, between the tendons of the flexor longus digitorum and flexor longus hallucis. Frictions over the nerve in this position give the same tingling feeling as when the "funny bone" is struck. By slightly stretching and inverting the foot, we can follow the nerve to its division into internal and external plantar nerves, where strong frictions produce marked pain.

The external saphenous nerve lies superficially in the middle line of the calf. As it is a sensory nerve, we pass from below upward, while giving light vibrations.

The external popliteal is best found behind the head of the

fibula, and frictions at that spot often produce a sparkling feeling in the foot.

Nervus Cruralis Anterior.

We can easily find this nerve where it lies in Scarpa's triangle, and apply frictions to it. Passing from it downward and toward the inner side of the thigh and knee, is the internal saphenous, which is purely sensory, and is therefore more effectively acted upon by vibrations in the centripetal direction.

Nervus Cutaneus Externus.

Sometimes neuralgic pains are felt in this branch of the lumbar plexus. We find the nerve about an inch below the anterior superior spine of the ilium.

Nervus Obturatorius.

In order to affect this nerve, we must flex and somewhat adduct the thigh. It passes out of the thyroid foramen at its upper border, and we must try to find it there.

Sensory Nerves on the Foot.

Coming forward below the external malleolus, we can easily follow the external saphenous, as it goes about half an inch or more above the outer edge of the foot.

The other sensory branches on the dorsum of the foot are derived from the external cutaneous and the terminal of the anterior tibial, the latter emerging between the first and second toe. We can stimulate these by simply passing quickly with the back of the nail transversely over the surface.

NERVES OF THE UPPER EXTREMITY.

We can reach all the chords of the brachial plexus either just above the clavicle at the base of the posterior triangle of the neck, and make frictions from before backward, or we may abduct the arm slightly, and pass our fingers high up into the axilla, and manipulate them there.

NERVUS CIRCUMFLEXUS.

The nerve passes through the quadrilateral space formed by the two teres muscles with the humerus and the long head of the triceps muscle, and, diving below the deltoid, it comes round the neck of the humerus. The arm is slightly abducted. We feel for the head of the humerus in the axilla, and ascertain the exact situation of the neck of the bone. The fingers are held as shown in Fig. 38, and the frictions are made from above downward, the same precautions as regards intervening tissues being taken here as elsewhere.

NERVUS MEDIANUS.

How this nerve is found I have already described (page 616). We can easily follow it in its whole course in the upper arm;

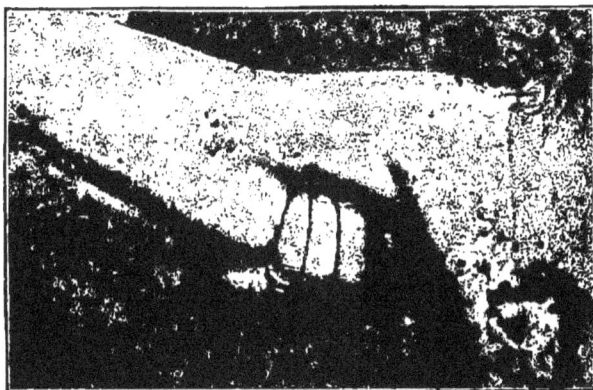

FIG. 42.

but in trying to reach it below the bend of the elbow, we must flex the arm somewhat, as the strong fascia in front of the elbow prevents us from coming down on it.

It lies to the inner side of the biceps muscle, being separated from it by the artery. The tips of the fingers are placed just inside the tendon, and the friction made from without inward.

NERVUS MUSCULO-SPIRALIS.

The place to find this nerve is where it emerges from under the outer head of the triceps muscle and in its course down between the brachialis anticus and the supinator longus (Fig. 43).

It is necessary first to abduct the arm, and then to somewhat flex the forearm toward the upper, because otherwise
we are unable to find the nerve, if our patient is a little mus-

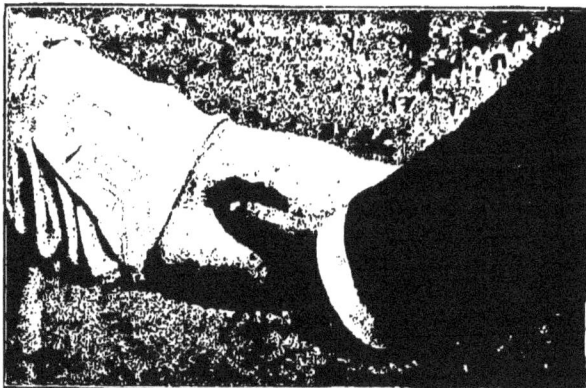

Fig. 43.

cular.   The frictions are best made with the last phalanx of
the thumb.   The feeling of tingling which the patient perceives
in the thumb, and even on the back of the hand, indicates a
correct friction.

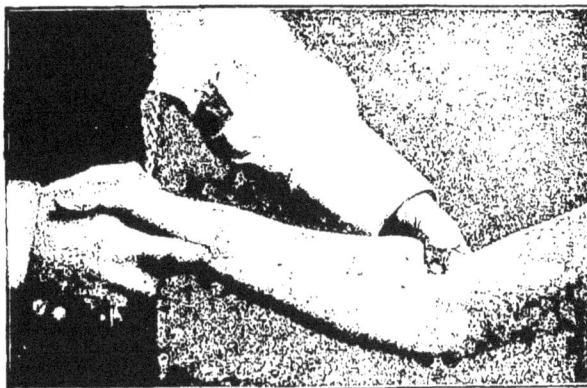

Fig. 44.

NERVUS RADIALIS.

This branch, the sensory continuation of the musculo-spiral
nerve, may be acted upon just below the bend of the elbow.

The arm is bent in order to relax the supinator longus muscle. The last phalanx of the thumb is placed at the inner border of that muscle and insinuated a little underneath it (Fig. 44).

At the same time as we quickly pronate the patient's forearm, we make the friction outward with the thumb. This goes under the muscle and over the nerve.

NERVUS POSTERIOR INTEROSSEUS OF THE MUSCULO-SPIRALIS.

We must first find the head of the radius. About an inch lower down, and between the radius and ulna, friction or pressure produces distinct strong pain, which is felt down to the wrist.

NERVUS ULNARIS.

We must feel for this nerve where it lies in the groove behind the internal condyle of the humerus. The high bony

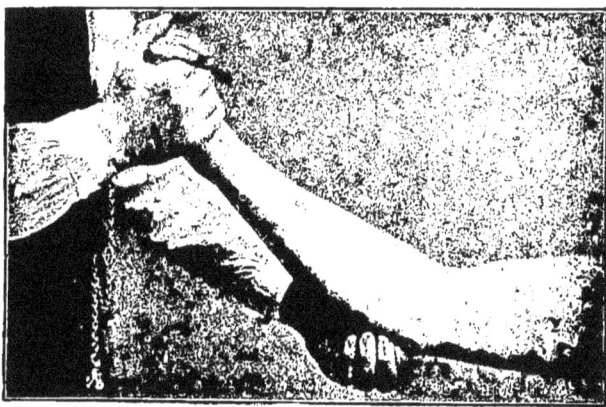

FIG. 45.

edges here somewhat prevent the application of a good friction. Therefore I always give it just underneath, where the nerve lies quite free (Fig. 45).

In this case it is also better to bend the arms slightly. The tingling in the little and the ring fingers corresponds in this, as in the other nerves of the arm, exactly to its distribution.

In the hand we once more meet with the median nerve.

It comes out just below the lower edge of the anterior annular ligament, where the nerve divides into its digital branches, and

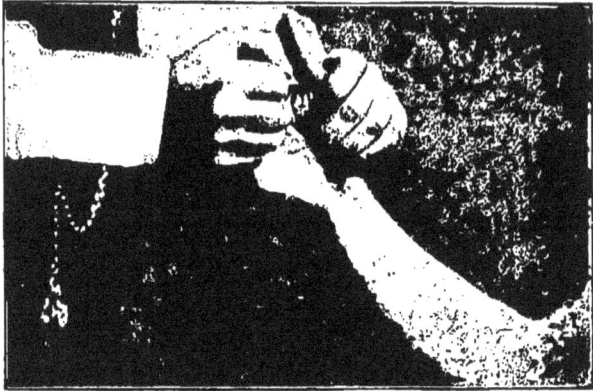

FIG. 46.

sends off the five **muscular** twigs. The patient's hand must be flexed. Fig. 46 shows how the friction or pressure is applied. It is felt very strongly indeed.

CHAPTER X.

PASSIVE EXTENSION OF THE MUSCLES.

THE passive extension is carried to the natural limit of the muscle, and is a passing, not a continued one. The stretching causes compression of the blood-vessels, while the nerves and the muscles are directly stimulated. After the completion of the movement, there will be an afflux of blood, and, following upon this, brisker nutritive changes. It has long been known that, if a muscle is stretched within certain limits, and not for too long a time, it becomes more sensitive to other mechanical stimulation, and contracts with greater force. In using Ling's exercises, it is therefore generally the custom to precede an active movement with passive extension, and to keep up the extension during the movement. In applying it, it is often found that apparently powerless muscles are capable of reacting against slight resistance, sometimes at once, sometimes after only a short treatment.

This passive extension stands on the borderland between passive and active movements, and at the commencement of treatment in many cases it is substituted for the latter, until strength begins to return in the affected muscles.

The expression "to keep up the extension during the movement" may seem a little extraordinary at first sight, and therefore I will try to explain it.

Suppose we have the movements of adduction and abduction of the upper arm, the patient resisting during the former, the manipulator during the latter. The shoulder-joint is the centre round which the movement takes place; the upper arm is the radius, with the elbow as the terminal point. (The forearm is supposed to be kept bent toward the upper one.) The manipulator, standing behind the patient, grasps his elbow, depresses it and stretches downward at the same time. Of course, in order to be able to do this, he does not hold his own arm at a right angle to that of the patient, but more in the same line with it. When now the abduction begins, he does not change the respective positions of the arms to each other, or at least very slightly, but makes the resistance not at a right angle, but at a smaller one. The smaller the angle, the stronger is the extension during the movement, and the more are the muscles stimulated to contraction.

There is another reason, and an important one, why we should make it a rule, when the joint is at all affected, to use passive extension in all movements, whether passive or active under resistance. By doing so, we remove the surfaces from each other, the friction is thus lessened, and the movement which under ordinary circumstances would cause considerable pain, can be given without any; it is also greater in range, and no irritation ensues.

CHAPTER XI.

THESE movements are rolling (circumduction), extension, flexion at different joints, etc. They are particularly used to diminish stiffness and to break down adhesions, etc., in joints; but it is likewise clear that they will also act more or less on the circulation, in accordance with the position the limb or part of it has while moving, and on the intermittent extension and relaxation of the veins, lymphatics, and capillary vessels in the muscles. Take, for instance, rolling of the leg (Fig. 52). If we make this movement slowly, the blood is gradually pumped toward the heart; but as the rapidity of the exercise increases, the stream quickens, the muscles are stimulated, a greater activity in the tissue interchange is produced, etc., and we have an action nearly as strong as if an active movement were made.

When pain in the joint is present, or if the patient is affected with heart disease, quickness is, of course, contra-indicated, but not otherwise. It is necessary to have the joint at which the movement takes place well under command. This is done either by the position the patient assumes, or by the hands of the manipulator. If not attended to, the movement cannot be well carried out and regulated; it becomes uncertain, and injury may be caused.

As the position of the patient and the application of the manipulator's hands are the same, or nearly so, in passive as in active extensions and flexions under resistance, with the exception of those for the head, I shall describe them along with these exercises, and confine myself here to a few rolling and some general movements for the head.

ROLLING OF THE HEAD.

The patient sits, and the operator stands at the side of him. One hand is placed on the forehead, the other below the occiput. The head rests in the latter, which is kept nearly immovable, while the former executes the movement. The

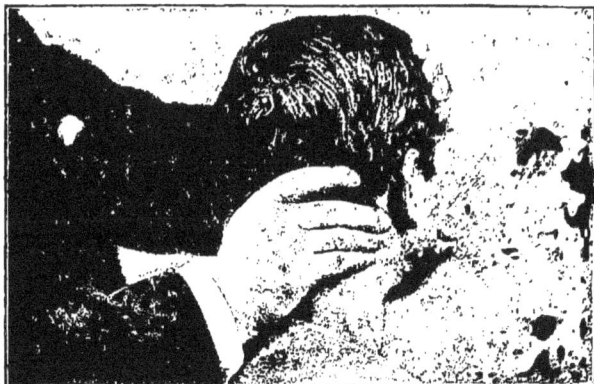

Fig. 47.

hand placed under the occiput confines the movement almost entirely to the occipito-atlantal joint (Fig. 47).

Turning the Head from Side to Side, and Bending it Forward.

The hands have much the same position as for circumduction (Fig. 48). During the side movements both hands are

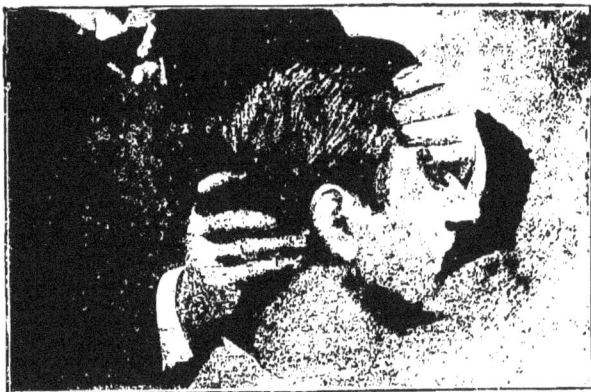

Fig. 48.

equally active, while during the one in the mesial plane, the posterior hand is principally used. Before the head is bent forward it is slightly inclined backward. In both movements the hand on the forehead makes light vibrations. These help to accelerate the flow of blood from the head.

In all these movements the head is lifted up—well seen in Fig. 48—before the exercise commences.

The object of them is to draw the blood from the head, as well as to diminish stiffness in the neck, as, for instance, from rheumatism. They are preceded by pétrissage or nerve vibrations, as the case may require.

ROLLING AT THE SHOULDER-JOINTS.

The patient sits, while the operator stands behind him, and if the joint is in any way affected, the patient's back is completely steadied.

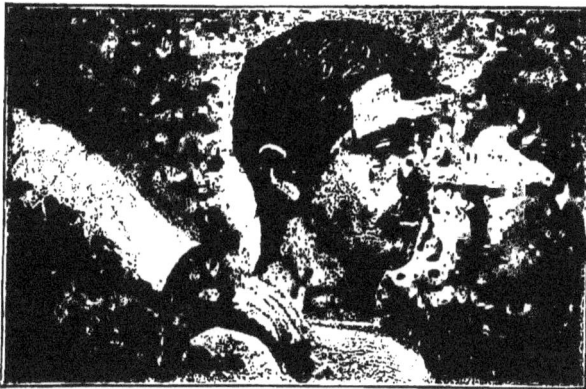

FIG. 40.

One hand is placed on the shoulder, the other below the elbow, as shown in Figs. 49 and 50.

The hand on the shoulder acts as a guard, and we can thus —say immediately after a dislocation has been reduced—give this exercise without any danger of the head of the humerus sliding out again. Then, also, when the bone is to be replaced, we press the fingers or the thumb on its head, and guide it on its course.

The movement may form part of a general treatment. The patient then sits unsupported on a low stool. The operator places one knee between the shoulders, in order to press the chest forward, and thus produce greater expansion of it, and deeper respiration during the movement.

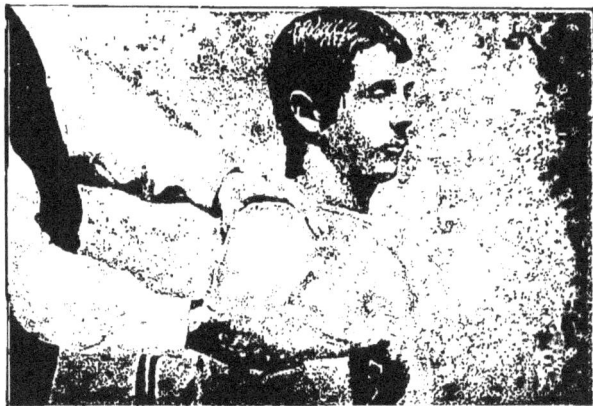

FIG. 50.

The patient's hands are grasped as in Fig. 63, and the elbows during such circumduction are carried well back.

Both arms are rolled at the same time.

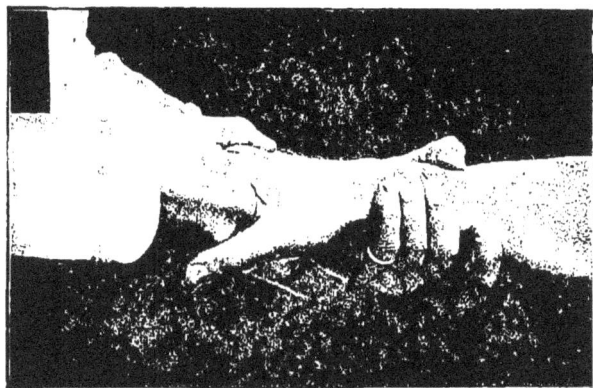

FIG. 51.

ROLLING AT THE WRIST-JOINTS.

The operator, standing in front of the patient, grasps with one hand the forearm just above the wrist, while with the other he takes hold of the patient's hand, as shown in Fig. 51, which also demonstrates very well the strong extension made before the beginning of the movement.

ROLLING AT THE HIP-JOINT.

The patient lies in the recumbent position, or half so. With one hand we grasp the heel, the wrist and forearm passing along the sole of the foot. The other, which steadies the

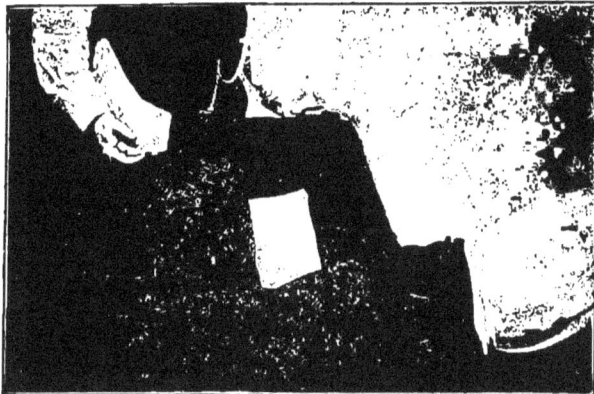

FIG. 52.

knee-joint, is placed on the knee, a little to the outer side (Fig. 52)

The hand on the foot executes the movement, while the other acts as a guide.

If the hip-joint alone is to be acted upon, the circumduction need not be so wide in its range; but should we wish to affect the knee-joint as well, or if given for the leg in general, then there must be complete extension at the knee-joint between each individual rolling.

ROLLING AT THE ANKLE-JOINT.

The patient's leg is so placed over the operator's knee, that the ankle-joint comes just over it. If now we grasp the malleoli with one hand, it is clear that we have complete control over the joint. The second hand makes the rolling, having the position on the foot shown in Fig. 53.

6

Fig. 54 shows where we apply our fingers when passive movements are made at the metacarpo-phalangeal joints. If, instead of taking hold of the forefingers by the first phalanx,

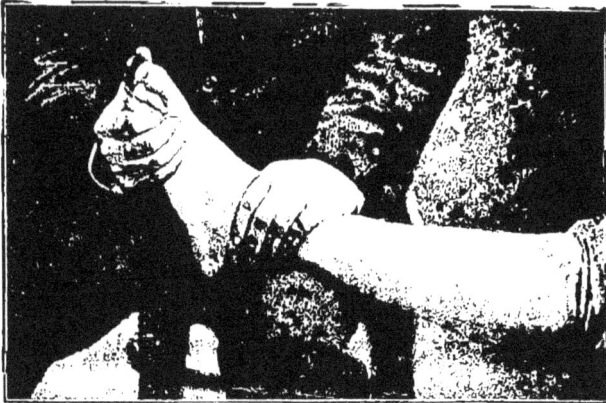

Fig. 53.

we grasped it by the tip, we would then have two intervening joints uncommanded, and this would be a great weakness and disadvantage.

The number of times these movements must be made,

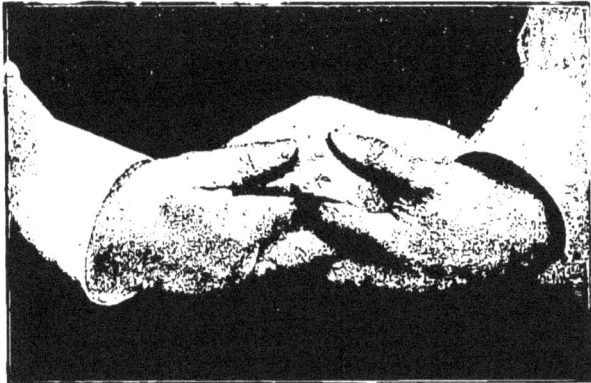

Fig. 54.

varies with the part, and also with the condition of the joints. It will be apparent that we cannot roll the head round as many times as an arm or leg, and the latter not so frequently in acute as in chronic affections, or when the rolling forms part of a general treatment.

Whenever we use these circumduction exercises, or extension and flexion, we must always carry out each individual movement to the utmost possible limit, exception being made in the instance of the head.

CHAPTER XII.

ACTIVE MOVEMENTS.

"MUSCLES are most perfect machines, but they are distinguished from all machines of human manufacture by the fact that by frequent exercise they become stronger, and are thereby capable of accomplishing more work" (Dubois Reymond).

When a muscle contracts, the veins and lymphatics are necessarily compressed, and more or less emptied, while as soon as the muscle relaxes there is an increased flow of oxygenated blood into it, and in consequence greater nourishment and growth of the existing muscular fibres; and if the contraction is repeated time after time, taking care, of course, that it is always kept within physiological limits, so that the muscle is not exhausted, a development of new muscular fibres takes place.

As a consequence of these two processes, the muscle becomes stronger and capable of doing more work.

All active movements have the effect of building up and strengthening the tissues.

But at the same time that the active movements have a local action, they have also a general influence.

It is evident that, having a given amount of blood in the body, when an increased flow to one part takes place, there must be a corresponding decrease of blood in the other parts of the body. It is for this purpose we use the active movements, viz., to produce metastasis.

As already stated, the active movements may be—

1. Free, *i.e.*, movements executed by the patient without any external help whatever.

2. Bound, *i.e.*, movements made either while steadiness and isolation are secured by apparatus, or under resistance.

Those made under resistance are again subdivided into—

(*a*) Those in which the operator resists.

(*b*) Those in which the patient resists.

The second group of movements, as can readily be understood, may be made to alternate for the same muscles, as for instance in the case of flexion and extension of the forearm on the upper, when the operator makes resistance to the bending and the patient to the stretching of the forearm.

It is necessary, before the commencement of each movement, that the patient should take up a correct position. By that I do not only mean a position in which the exercise can be best executed, but also one in which the chest is free, while deep and steady respiration must be kept up. In the movements, for instance, with the arms, depicted in Figs. 62 and 63, the respiration must be so regulated that deep inspiration is made when the arms are separated from the chest, and expiration when they are again approximated to it, because in the former case the chest is expanded, in the latter its capacity is diminished.

Simultaneously with the quickening of the circulation, a greater amount of blood is sent to the lungs, carrying with it more carbonic acid; and the need for oxygen in the body is greater, thus necessitating stronger and deeper respiration.

Indeed, a correct position is nearly of as much importance as the movement itself.

Every active exercise must be made, or given, slowly, exception being taken in those movements by which we desire, through their very rapidity, to influence the circulation. After the completion of a movement—say stretching of the arms— the patient remains for a few seconds with them in that position, in order that as great an effect as possible may be produced.

We must also bear in mind that the muscular power is strongest at the middle, smallest at the beginning and end, of the movement; and therefore the resistance must be graduated, and must increase and decrease with the increase and decrease of the muscular power.

In the free active movements, there is little or no isolation of the muscles, but in the bound ones we can, of course, localize them as much as we like.

The active movements are usually repeated three or four times.

I now pass on to describe a few of these exercises.

1. FREE.

BENDING FORWARD AND RAISING OF THE TRUNK, WITH THE ARMS STRETCHED UP.

The patient either stands with his feet together, or he has them apart a distance of twenty to twenty-four inches, as in the illustration, in order to secure a broader base, and with it more steadiness in the movement. The arms are stretched

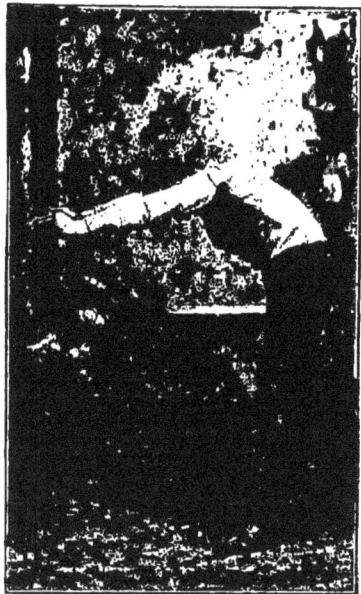

FIG. 55.

straight up, the distance between the hands corresponding to the transverse diameter of the chest.

Before the movement begins, the patient stretches himself to the very utmost, and then he slowly bends forward. The back is not to be kept straight while he does so, because all the segments of the vertebral column then become immovable, and the movement which takes place is from the very beginning greatest at the hip-joint, and we have, so to speak, only a falling forward of the trunk. The exercise must, on the contrary, begin at the upper part of the spinal column, and gradually pass down vertebra after vertebra; and on raising the trunk again, it is at the lower part of the back that the move-

ment begins and passes as gradually upward. In this way the
muscular slips of the deeper muscles of the back come fully
into play, and they act like so many elastic strings, which,
having the weight (the head and arms) at the upper end, and
a fixed point below from which their band action starts, must,
when the movement goes forward, necessarily extend the spine
more completely, and in a case of lateral curvature of the
back also rotate the vertebræ. The patient has then to try to
keep as much as possible in the mesial plane, in order that the
elongated tongues of the relaxed muscles may come more
effectively in action.

The patient on rising up does not stop at the erect position,
but goes somewhat backward, partly in order to get a deeper
inspiration, partly to exercise the abdominal muscles, and in
this manner to get equality between the antagonists.

A very simple, but none the less effective respiratory movement is this: The patient stands completely erect, with the
arms down to the sides. He now makes the following exercise: He carries the arms slowly forward and upward, always
maintaining the proper distance between the hands, and when
they are in the vertical position he draws them backward by
bringing the muscles of the shoulders more strongly into
play. Slowly as they were carried up, they are now taken
downward and outward. As the arms are raised from the
sides, the chest becomes more and more expanded. The
patient has to make deep inspiration while the movement pro-
gresses toward its climax, and afterward makes gradual expiration. This movement, when well executed, is felt very strongly
in the shoulder muscles. It is therefore also indicated for
those whose shoulders have a tendency to fall forward, as
well as for chronic disorders of the lungs.

II. BOUND.

A. With Help of Apparatus.

BENDING BACKWARD AT THE UPPER PART OF THE BACK.

The patient stands at a distance somewhat less than the
length of his own foot from the wall. He places his hands on
his hips, with his elbows well thrown back. Then he stretches
himself and bends backward. When the movement cannot
be continued any further, the patient falls back until the back

of his head touches the wall by which he stands (Fig. 56).
Then he slowly rises up on his toes, and while doing so draws
a deep inspiration and goes slowly down again.

The movement does not take place in the lumbar region at
all, but higher up between the shoulders. We have to do with
movable rings, each formed by a vertebra and a pair of ribs.
As now the spinal processes are by the backward bending,
small as it is, approximated to each other, the freer segments

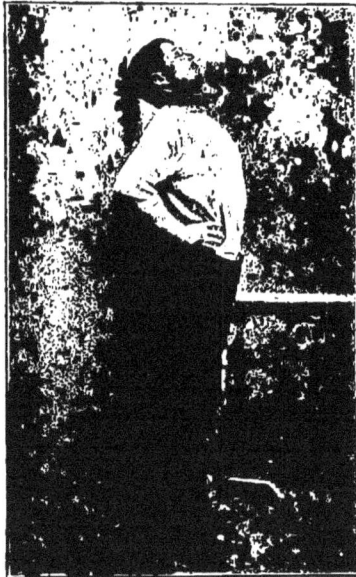

Fig. 56.

of the rings must come further away and widen the inter-
spaces. The chest becomes greatly expanded, and the exercise
is thus a powerful respiratory movement.

STRETCHING AND BENDING OF THE KNEE.

The patient places one foot against the seat of a chair, and
with his hands he takes hold of the back of it (Fig. 57). The
correct position, however, is with the arms straight forward
from the shoulders, and with the hands grasping some fixed
object at the same level. Why should the arms be stretched
horizontally forward? Because the patient then stands erect,
and we have the normal distance between the two attach-
ments of the hamstring muscles. In Fig. 57 this distance is

increased because of the bending forward. As we see, this
may serve as a position in which to give tapotement of the
perineum, sacral and gluteal regions. The operator, while
giving this tapotement, stands on the opposite side to that of
the raised leg. In such a case, therefore, as represented in
Fig. 57, he would take up his position on the left side.

When the knee-joint is stiff, he must be on the same side as
the affected limb. The patient has to stretch the leg to the

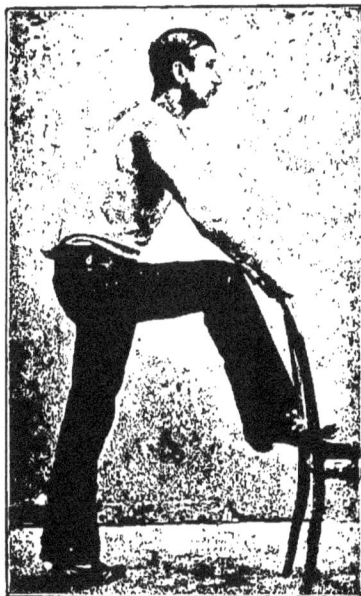

FIG. 57.

utmost of his ability, and when he has reached the limit, we
produce a greater extension at the knee-joint by laying one
hand on it, placing the other below the buttock, and by drawing backward we extend passively the hamstring muscles, at
the same time as the hand on the knee presses it down. I
have often seen a knee stretched completely straight, where
from stiffness in the muscles the patient himself was entirely
unable to effect this movement.

The patient keeps it extended for a little, and then he bends
it until thigh and leg are at least at right angles to each
other, and complete relaxation of the muscles is produced.
Sometimes, of course, we must begin with the foot, quite low
down at the floor, and gradually work upward as the patient

improves, until he can straighten his knee, when the foot is placed at the same height as the hip-joint.

The action on the muscles, blood-vessels, and nerves on the posterior part of the thigh and leg—particularly on the former —is very great. The effect of the movement, especially on the muscles of the calf, is much increased by depressing the heel after the knee has been extended.

The limb on which the patient stands must be kept completely straight, otherwise the exercise loses a good deal of its effect.

This movement is more especially used in contraction of the hamstring muscles and those of the calf, stiffness and other affections of the knee-joint, in sciatica, and also for the general circulation.

EXTENSION OF THE MUSCLES OF THE CALF.

If, standing with the legs straight, we make strong dorsiflexion of the foot, the muscles of the calf are extended, and

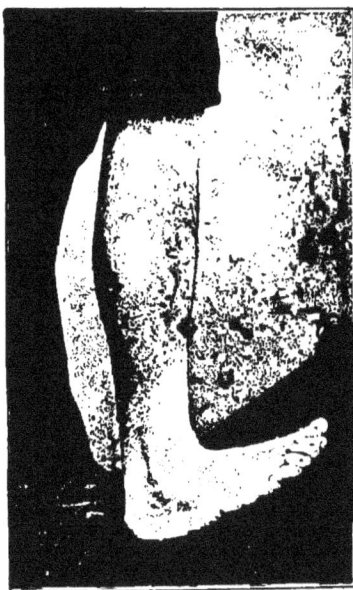

FIG. 58.

the movement goes on until it is stopped, partly by the wedging of the astragalus between the malleoli, and partly by the band action of the muscles of the calf. We can increase the intensity of this movement by placing the foot against, say, a wall at an angle of 45°, or on something situated at the same angle, and then with straight knee moving the whole body forward (Fig. 58). The extension is felt very strongly in the muscles of the calf. If the knee is bent, the movement loses its effect, because the points of attachment of the muscles become approximated to each other.

The movement is mostly employed for muscular and nervous stimulations, and for stiffness in the ankle-joint.

RAISING OF THE LEGS OR TRUNK WHILE LYING ON THE BACK (Figs. 59, 60).

We have here two movements shown in full action, in which the psoas and iliacus muscles take the principal part,

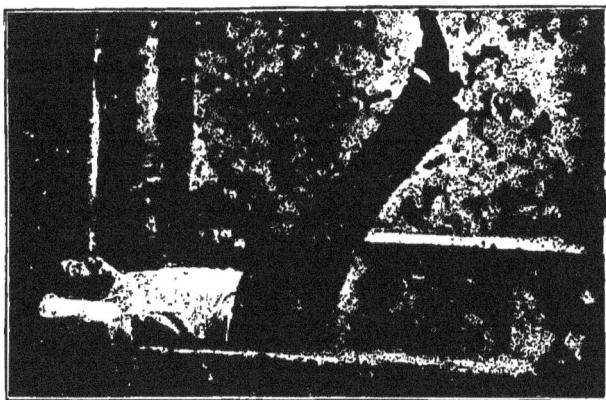

FIG. 59.

but in which the muscles of the lower extremities are also at work—only the fixed point is reversed. The primary position for the patient is to lie straight on his back. In Fig. 59 he lifts the legs up to a right angle or more. In Fig. 60 he gradually raises the trunk until he attains a sitting position. In the exercise depicted in Fig. 59 we sometimes steady the patient by laying our hands on the elbows, while in the raising of the trunk the hands grasp the ankles; and in both we isolate the psoas and iliacus muscles by deep abdominal respiration.

That full respiration is necessary we can readily understand, for the muscles of the lower extremity are more or less
in action, keeping the knee and ankle steady, so that the psoas
and iliacus may have an immovable attachment from which
to start their action.   In doing so, they for the time compress
the vessels, and the blood is largely driven out of the limbs.
If now, as so often happens, the patient holds his breath, the
blood does not pass so well into the lungs, and the abdominal
muscles adding their pressure, the right side of the heart gets
overfilled with venous blood.   Thus we have also backward
pressure in the vessels of the head and neck.

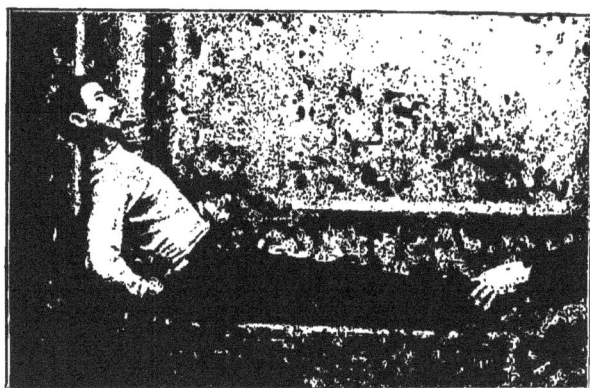

Fig. 60.

The movements are made very slowly, and in both we
make the patient stop at different angles to the plane in which
he lies.   This greatly increases the muscular work.

We can, in the movement shown in Fig. 60, augment the
work by folding the hands behind the neck, and again by
having the arms stretched straight up.   The patients, when
they begin to feel tired of continuing the exercise, have a habit
of drawing the shoulders forward and thus pressing the chest
together.   This is on no account to be allowed.

These exercises are to be used in weakness and pain in the
lumbar region.   They also act on the organs in the abdominal
cavity.

In the position the patient occupies in Fig. 59, a movement
acting on the adductor muscles of the thigh can easily be
made simply by letting the legs slowly fall outward as far as

possible from one another, and then by as slowly approximating them again.

Extension of Back in the Prone Position.

In Fig. 61 we see a movement which acts especially on the muscles of the back, but also on those on the posterior aspect of the lower extremity. The patient lies in the prone position, with the hands steadied at the hips, the fingers forward and the thumbs backward. If they are reversed, they necessitate the carrying forward of the shoulders, and with that compression of the chest. On the contrary, the shoulders are to be

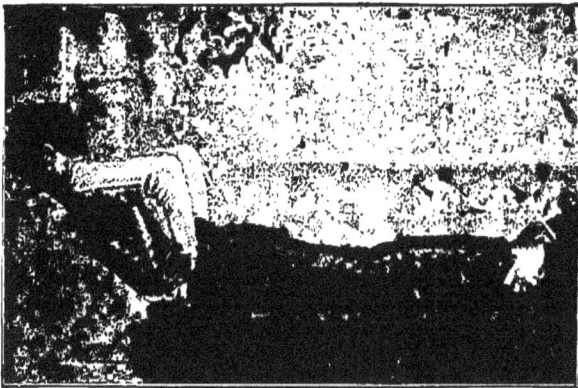

Fig. 61.

well thrown back and deep inspiration made, as it is not only a movement for the back, but, secondarily, also for the chest.

It is used after tapotement of the back, or alone as a muscular stimulation, and in a general treatment.

As the patient gets accustomed to the exercise, the hands are applied to the neck, or extended straight forward parallel with the ears.

B. Made under Resistance either from Patient or Operator.

Bending and Stretching of the Neck.

The patient stands quite erect, with his hands steadied against the wall of the room. The operator places his hands well below the base of the patient's head, having the thenar part of the palm on each side behind the mastoid process, and

the thumbs lying horizontally under the occiput. The patient
now makes resistance while the operator bends the head
forward, after having first well stretched the neck (Fig.
62). When the movement reaches its anterior limit, the
patient in his turn raises the head, the manipulator making
resistance.

Through this movement the muscles of the back of the
neck in general are affected, but the influence of its action is
also felt at the upper part of the back. If we wish to isolate
the movement to one side of the neck, say for instance in
rheumatism of the right side, the patient turns his face to the

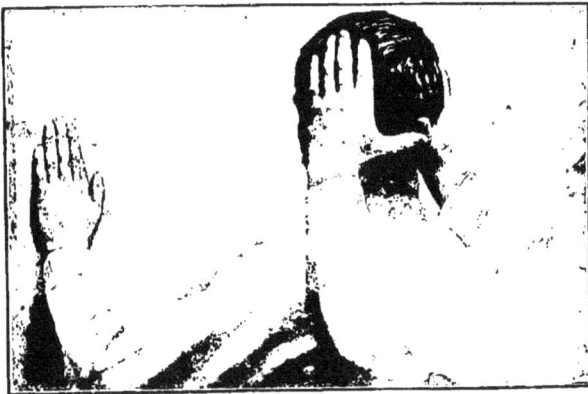

Fig. 62.

right and inclines it backward. We then use only one hand,
and place the other on the opposite side to act as a guard
during the manipulation.

Carrying the Arms Forward and Backward in the Horizontal Plane.

The patient may sit with his back steadied or stand free.
He extends the arms forward, with the normal distance between the hands. If he stands, he must place one foot forward, the length of an ordinary step, for security of the
position. Made in this way the movement is considerably
stronger. The operator standing in front of him places his
hands as in Fig. 63.

The patient carries the arms back under resistance, and resists himself when the arms are brought forward by the operator.

As we see from the course of the movement, it acts more especially on the muscles passing between the shoulder-blades and the humerus, but since the rhomboid and trapezius muscles, starting from the spine, are nearly as much exerted in order to give the other muscles a steady point to work from, the action of the movement has a marked influence upon them too.

Made with both arms at the same time, it is distinctly a

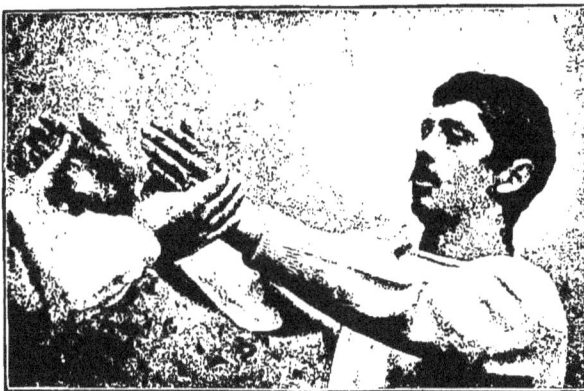

FIG. 63.

movement for the chest, by its action of drawing the shoulders back, and by that of lifting up the thorax. Made with one arm at a time, correction of the rotation in lateral curvatures of the spine is produced.

STRETCHING AND BENDING OF THE ARMS.

The patient sits on a low stool. The operator places his knee against the patient's back between the shoulders, partly to steady him, partly for expansion of the chest. Fig. 64 shows the grasp of the hands, the turning out of the elbows, and consequent throwing back of the shoulders. The patient stretches the arms straight up and draws them down again, the operator making resistance on both occasions.

At the same time that it is a movement for the arms, it also affects the chest by producing greater expansion.

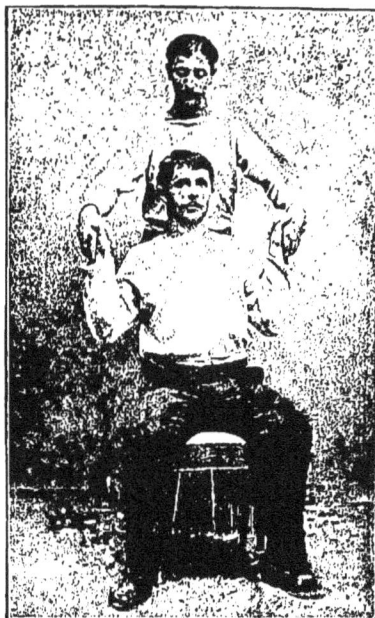

FIG. 64.

STRETCHING AND BENDING AT THE ELBOW-JOINT.

The patient sits or stands. With one hand we grasp the elbow, in order to command that joint, and with the other the hand and wrist, as seen in Fig. 65.

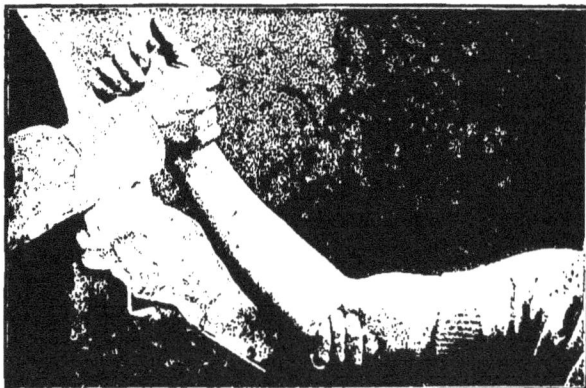

FIG. 65.

Here the movement is shown with the arm midway between supination and pronation, in order that the supinator longus muscle may more particularly be put in action. We make the resistance both at the bending and stretching, or the patient makes the resistance in both movements.

Used for stiffness of the elbow-joint, muscular stimulation, etc.

Stretching and Bending at the Knee-Joint.

The operator places the patient's knee above his own thigh, and lays one hand over that joint, and the other over the

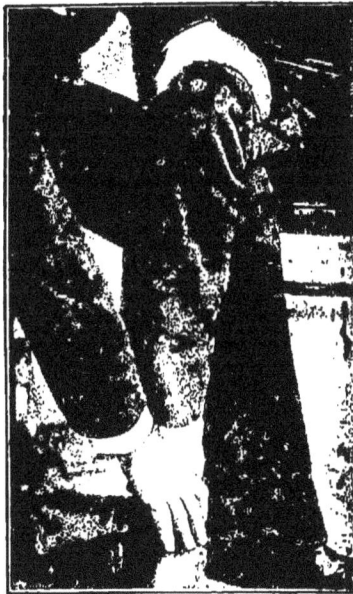

Fig. 66.

dorsum of the foot (Fig. 66). The patient extends and flexes his leg, while the operator makes resistance. During the flexion of the limb, the hand on the dorsum of the foot is placed behind the heel and ankle-joint.

Stretching of the Vertebral Column.

I cannot remember having seen this movement used in Stockholm, but my brother always employs it in curvatures of the spine.

7

The patient stands as erect as possible, with his back against the wall of the room (Fig. 67). The operator stands in front of him, and lays one hand on the patient's head, while with the other he steadies him. (The left hand in the figure is somewhat awkwardly placed.) He now presses downward, at the same time that the patient is told to stretch upward with all his might. The top of the column being thus fixed, the short deep muscles at the upper part of the back take

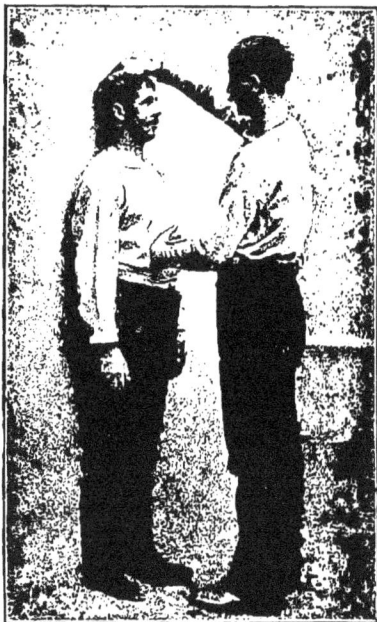

Fig. 67.

their steady point above, and so act from above downward while the lower ones work from below upward.

In a case of spinal curvature, the slips of the deeper dorsal muscles, which have become weakened and elongated, are thus brought into action. We must take care not to bend the head forward during the exercise, as the movement then entirely loses its effect, because the fixed point above is moved.

TURNING OF THE TRUNK IN THE SITTING POSTURE.

The patient sits on a low stool. Either he must have the feet fixed by some means, or an assistant must steady his knees; otherwise the movement is not confined to the trunk. He has the hands folded behind the neck, sits with his back completely straight, and with the head well back. The operator applies his hands to the patient's elbows (Fig. 68).

The movement now begins, the patient turning toward either side (the left in the figure), and resistance is made by the operator with the left hand behind and the right one in front. This resistance must be equal on both sides. When

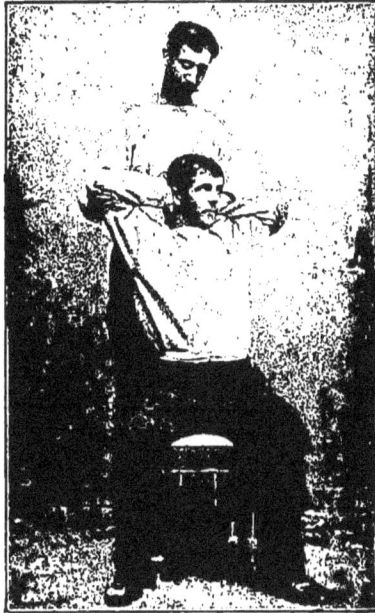

FIG. 68.

the patient has gone round as far as he can, he turns forward again, also under resistance, which, however, has changed, being in front on the left side and behind on the right. When he again sits with the face straight forward, a few seconds' rest is made, and the same repeated on the other side.

If we recall the arrangement of the muscles of the trunk, we shall understand how wide the effect of this exercise really is. Starting below at the crest of the ilium on the right, the fibres of the external oblique of the abdomen pass upward and backward. In the region of the thorax this same direction is maintained by the external intercostal muscles; still further back there is a similar arrangement in the short fibres which constitute the great oblique rotator muscles of the spine; and we must also remember that in front we have the internal oblique and internal intercostals on the left side whose fibres run in the same direction as those of the external muscles of the right.

Besides using the exercise for circulatory purposes and for the muscles, we have recourse to it in different intestinal affections.

It will be clear that we can also give passive movements to the patient going in the same direction and with the same application of the hand, in all the above positions, except the stretching of the back.

LIFTING OF THE LEG WHILE LYING ON THE SIDE.

In Fig. 69 we see the position the patient takes up before the exercise begins. Fig. 70 shows how the movement is made under resistance. The operator stands with his side

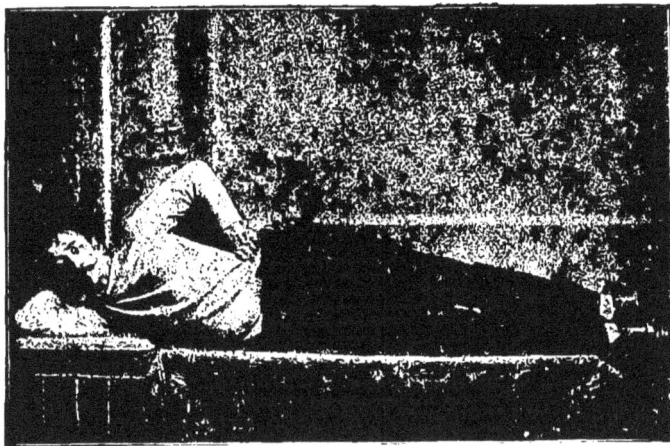

FIG. 69.

against the patient, steadying him at the gluteal region. With one hand he grasps the heel and ankle in such a manner that the thumb lies parallel to the outer border of the foot. The other hand is placed on the knee. The patient, holding the leg completely straight, lifts it slowly up in the middle line as high as he can, while the operator makes resistance. The latter afterward presses it down, the patient resisting. If we

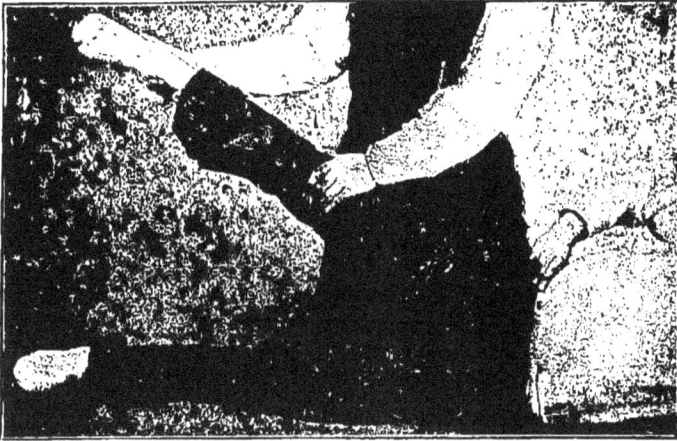

Fig. 70.

carry the foot a little backward or a little forward, we bring the anterior and the posterior parts of the muscular mass in the gluteal region into play to a greater extent.

ABDUCTION OF THE KNEES (Fig. 71).

The patient lies in the semi-recumbent position, the knees being bent and the feet resting at the same level as the buttocks. The operator stands in front of the patient, and places one hand on the outer side of each knee. The patient abducts the thigh under resistance from the operator, and the latter afterward adducts the knees while the patient resists. In this way the abductors of the thighs are strongly acted upon. One must stand in front of the patient in order to produce extension of the muscles.

In the same position the adductor muscles of the thighs can also be exercised if resistance be made on the inner side of the knees when they are approximated to each other, or if the operator adducts the knees, the patient making resistance.

The intensity of the movements is increased when the patient sits on a high bench with the back steadied and the legs stretched out. The operator's hands are then applied on

the feet instead of the knees. The increased length of the
lever increases the muscular work for the patient, while at

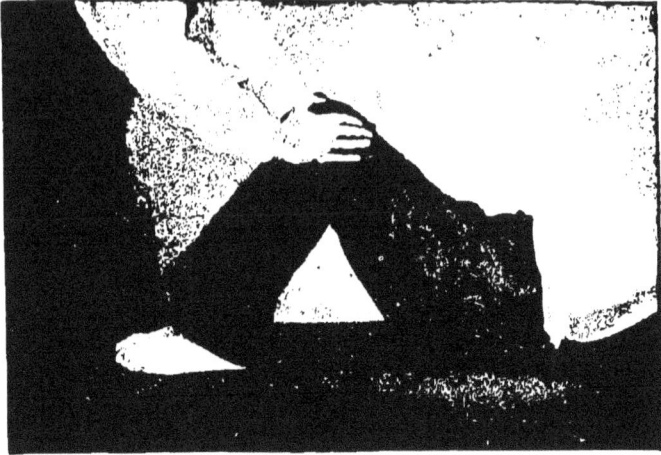

FIG. 71.

the same time it lessens the force necessary to be exerted
by the operator.

CHAPTER XIII.

CASES ILLUSTRATING THE TREATMENT.

I. PAROTITIS BILATERALIS.

ARTILLERYMAN N. was taken under treatment on the 17th of December, 1888.

The parotid glands on both sides were swollen, the swelling extending from the zygomatic arch to below the lower jaw. They were hard and painful, and had the size of a hen's egg. The pain was so great that the patient was unable to open his mouth. Hearing impaired. The illness commenced on the previous day.

Progress.—After about twenty minutes' treatment, the glands sank to within a third of their former volume, and were soft.

December 18th. Pain and swelling less than after treatment the day before.

December 19th. Hears well again; no pain, no swelling; movement of lower jaw painless and free.

Treatment.—Pétrissage. The pressure was applied in a half circle, from above backward and downward. I stood behind the patient, and used the ball of the thumbs, in order that no unnecessary pain should be caused. The pétrissage did not act quickly enough, and therefore vibrations were made with the same parts of my hands, which had a greater effect in diminishing not only the pain, but also the swelling. I also gave frictions over the facial nerve for about a minute.

II. TONSILLITIS.

Rinaldo N., 22 years old, non-commissioned officer of the I. and R. Navy, came for treatment on the 11th December, 1888.

Both tonsils began to swell the day before. They were now covered with pus. On the right side, the pus coverings extended over wide areas, while on the left side they formed several smaller points. The tonsils themselves were very swollen, and difficulty and pain were experienced in swallowing.

Progress.—After the treatment the patient felt better. The difficulty of swallowing was greatly lessened.

December 12th. Tonsils much smaller. The pus coverings have disappeared on both sides.

December 13th. The tonsils are very nearly normal. No difficulty or pain in deglutition. Treated for the last time.

Treatment.—The patient was subjected to treatment for fifteen minutes each day. It consisted in the two movements for the throat shown in Figs. 20 and 23, the former for five, the latter for about ten minutes, and frictions over the facial nerve separately; but it is clear that the manipulation behind the ascending ramus of the lower jaw stimulates the nerve the whole time, since the fingers pass over it continually.

III. TONSILLITIS.

Rezic, 28 years old, maid-servant, residing at Trieste, had taken cold on the first day of her menstrual period, the 22d of January, 1889. On that day and during the night, fever, with shivering, difficulty of and pain in swallowing, set in. She also suffered from a severe headache.

She was under the care of Dr. Michele Brown, the distinguished specialist for diseases of the nose, throat, and larynx.

I myself was under his treatment at Trieste. He mentioned the case to me on the morning of the 23d, and asked if I would treat her, and thus illustrate to him the way in which I gave the manipulations for the throat.

The patient's temperature was 39° C. She shivered and felt cold, and had great pain in swallowing; both tonsils were inflamed, each with a continuous white covering, more especially on the right side. The skin was dry and hot, the head ached very much, and the lymphatic glands were enlarged.

Progress and Treatment.—January 23d. I gave the shakings as shown in Figs. 20–23 for about five minutes each, and the pain and difficulty of swallowing passed nearly away; also frictions for three minutes in the neck, more particularly over the second pair of cervical nerves. The patient felt the cold sensation, which nearly always accompanies administration of these frictions, very strongly. The shivering ceased, she turned warm, and the skin moist. This was followed by general pétrissage of the abdomen.

In the evening at six o'clock the temperature was 38.6° C.; pulse, 132. Same treatment as in the morning. The pulse immediately went down to 96. She now also told me that she had severe pains in the sacral region, and that she had had them very strongly at the menstrual periods since the time, six months previously, when she had a child. I gave nerve frictions over the sacrum, with the consequence that the pain entirely passed away.

January 24th. Not treated in the morning. The pain on swallowing had diminished considerably. Up to ten o'clock the evening before, she had felt well, but at that hour the fever set in again.

Dr. Brown took the temperature an hour after the treatment the preceding night, and found it normal. This sudden effect astonished him, and he asked Dr. Escher and Dr. Gormond, the former surgeon and the latter physician to the Infirmary at Trieste, to be present at my next visit. We decided to treat the patient in the evening only at six o'clock.

The pulse had again risen to 122, and the temperature was 38° C. I gave the same treatment as the day before. The pain in the throat went entirely away. I gave the nerve frictions in the neck for two minutes. Dr. Escher and Dr. Gormond each took one hand, and felt the pulse during the frictions. They said that at first it changed, being sometimes slower, sometimes quicker, then it got more even, and at the expiration of the two minutes it went comparatively slowly, at the rate of 90 beats a minute.

An hour afterward the temperature was again normal. The patient felt easy and well; the pain at the small of her back remained away.

January 25th. The patient was well. No discomfort on swallowing. Tonsils no longer inflamed; the coverings gone. Temperature normal; pulse, 72. Treated for the last time.

IV. DIPHTHERIA.

Private Inc F. turned ill on the 10th of December, 1888, and was the same day removed to the Marine Infirmary.

On the 11th, at four o'clock in the afternoon, I saw him for the first time.

The tonsils were very much swollen—the right one most; they nearly met in the middle. The right tonsil was covered with a large gangrenous membrane; on the left the covering was smaller. The lymphatic and submaxillary glands were enlarged, especially on the right side, where they formed a large continuous swelling. Deglutition extremely painful. Temperature, 39.6° C.; pulse, 104.

Progress.—The treatment was begun at once. The swelling of the glands diminished visibly, and they turned softer. 9 P.M. The diffuse swelling is soft and œdematous. The patient complains that the sputum and fluids he drinks pass out through the nose. He keeps the mouth very open. Temperature, 38.7° C.; pulse, 92.

After the treatment the external swelling had nearly disappeared. Expectoration easier; he closes the mouth, and says he feels better.

December 13th. Morning temperature, 37.7° C. The swelling of the tonsil on the right side diminished, and the membranous covering smaller; the left side is also clearer.

December 14th. Membranous covering continues to diminish. Temperature, 37.3° C.

December 16th. Deglutition easier, but the fluids still pass out of his nose on drinking.

December 17th. On left tonsil the covering loosens; the tonsils much smaller; lymphatic glands normal.

December 20th. Pharyngeal surfaces normal. Patient well and convalescent.

On the 30th, the patient left the hospital, and went on three weeks' leave. He came back from this with paralytic symptoms. These spread, bulbar paralysis set in, and on the afternoon of the 2d of February, 1889, the patient died from paralysis of the heart—the very day I returned to Pola after a five weeks' absence.

V. DIPHTHERIA.

The girl Papic, 8 years old. On the 9th of December, 1888, the tonsils were red and swollen, and had a membranous covering.

December 10th. Membrane on both tonsils. Fever; glands swollen.

December 11th. The membranous covering spreading.

Progress.—December 12th. She came under my hands. The temperature, 37.7° C.; pulse, 110. She keeps the mouth open; breathing snoring, expression of face quiet. The tonsils very swollen, especially the left one, so that they nearly meet. The membranous covering passes on to the soft palate. The nose is free. On the left side the lymphatic glands are as large as hazel-nuts, on the right as almonds; the submaxillary glands are swollen—all are tender.

Evening, nine o'clock. Temperature, 37.4° C.; pulse, 92. Treated both in the morning and evening for about 20 minutes.

December 13th. Yesterday the membranous coverings were brushed away with lactic acid. To-day they are more continuous and thicker, and are spreading forward on the left side; on the right side, the covering shows on separate places. Since yesterday, the fluid she drinks passes through the nose. The glands on the right side are larger; on the left, œdematous swelling is present, especially in the submaxillary region.

Evening. Temperature, 37.6° C.; pulse, 102. During the treatment a great amount of saliva flows out of the mouth. After it, the girl feels easier, the glands are softer and smaller.

December 14th. Slept fairly well during the night. Morning temperature, 37.7° C.; evening, 37.8°.

December 15th. Evening, ten o'clock. Temperature, 37.6° C.; pulse, 108. Breathing very snoring. Nose is clogged up. Expression of face apathetic. Membranous covering on right side as before. On the left, it spreads thickly over the whole tonsil, over the soft palate and on to the uvula.

The pulse intermits sometimes (every fifth or sixth beat); is very small.

The breathing occasionally stops. After thirty minutes' treatment, the pulse was quieter and was regular; same with the respiration.

December 16th. Forenoon. Temperature, 36.7° C. Slept a little during the night, but snored very much. From the nose a great amount of thick stuff came out. Expression of face quiet; she takes an interest in the surroundings. Breathing free; the nose free.

Membranes on right side thrown off. Tonsil on the left less swollen; membrane contracted and lessened, split in the middle and at several places. The glands are much smaller. Treated 20 minutes.

December 17th. Morning. Temperature, 37° C. Slept well; no snoring after two o'clock. Perspired slightly during the night. Left tonsil free at the front; left palate near it the same; the covering on uvula loosens, same posteriorly; right tonsil clear.

Evening temperature, 37° C. Treated 25 minutes.

December 18th. Has slept well; plays and takes food with appetite. Temperature, 37.2° C. The membranous covering only present as small islands. The lymphatic and submaxillary glands are normal.

December 19th. Slept well. Œdema of the right inferior eyelid. Albumin in urine, 1%. Quantity of urine small. General condition yet continues good; she plays. Treatment 35 minutes. Œdema gone.

Evening. No œdema. The child plays and laughs.

December 20th. The remainder of the membrane on left side hangs free as a sail from the tonsil. Temperature, 37.6° C. Treated 35 minutes; the throat, 15 minutes; back and abdomen during the rest of the time.

December 21st. Urine has 1% albumin. Membrane completely gone. Treatment as before.

December 22d. Urine still contains albumin. Throat treated 10 minutes, with pétrissage of the abdomen. I also gave vibrations over the kidneys.

December 23d. Urine contains albumin in the proportion of about 1 to a thousand. Quantity greater. Child looks well.

December 24th. Quantity of urine about normal. Traces of albumin scarcely discernible.

Here I stopped the treatment. On the 6th of January, 1889, the patient was sent home.

Treatment.—The treatment is here the same as for angina (tonsillitis), only vibrations are at the beginning substituted for shakings, and the latter must be made much more delicately. The nerve frictions in the neck are continued for some minutes. The whole is to be concluded with general pétrissage of the abdomen, accompanied by nerve frictions over the dorsal sensory nerves.

In the case of the girl Papic, I gave on the first days of the appearance of albumin in the urine kneading of the kidneys. On the 22d I gave vibrations instead, and on the following day the quantity of urine was increased and the albumin diminished. The treatment in both cases lasted from twenty-five to thirty-five minutes, and the patients were treated twice a day.

VI. POST-DIPHTHERITIC PARALYSIS.

I treated the following case during the summer of 1887, at Leipsic, in the clinic of Dr. Moebius, the well-known authority on nervous diseases; and I have already recorded it in the medical press ("Medical Press and Circular," July 25th, 1888).

Mary A., aged 15, a native of Leipsic, was seized with diphtheria in the second week of December, 1886, and was for four weeks confined to her bed. On several occasions she was nearly choked, and her mother probably saved her life by tearing away large pieces (grosse Stücke weggerissen) with a spoon. A young member of the family, a boy, three years old, died of diphtheria at that time. The patient's progress toward recovery was very slow. She could not go out of doors until the middle of February, 1887. The soft palate remained paralyzed for a considerable time. Even in May and June regurgitation of food into the nose now and then occurred.

About the middle of May, the patient began to feel weakness in the legs, and consequently difficulty in walking. She was sent into the country, but returned after a fortnight in a worse condition. The weakness increased day by day, until at last she was quite unable to walk without assistance. Her doctor then advised her to consult Dr. Moebius, and she attended his clinic on the 23d of June, 1887. Her condition on that day, shortly stated, was as follows:

The patient looked pale and weak. Her appetite was not good. She was very nervous, and shed tears on the slightest provocation. Sensation in the feet, ankles, and lower parts of the legs was greatly impaired. The weakness in the legs was not preceded or accompanied by any pain. She could only take a few steps without help, and even these in a very waddling manner. She lost her balance in walking, and also when she closed her eyes.

When told to extend or bend her feet, she only succeeded in producing slight movements of the toes. The powers of

flexion and extension at the knee-joint were gone. Adduction
of the thighs could be performed with some exertion, while the
abductor muscles had almost lost their power. She required
assistance to rise from her chair, or while standing with her
feet wide apart to bend her body forward or sideways and
raise it up again; her inability being due partly to loss of
balance, partly to muscular weakness. The patellar reflex
was absent. Her sight had been affected, but the power of
accommodation was now normal. The voice had a slight nasal
twang, and, as said before, regurgitation of food into the nose
had sometimes occurred during the month. No electrical tests
were tried.

Progress.—From June 23d to July 2d I treated the patient
four times. By the latter date the sensation was greatly improved, and there was more strength in the back. The feet
had regained some power, but she was still unable to perform
the movements of eversion and inversion.

July 9th. The patient had received further four treatments. The sensation in feet and legs was completely restored. She could bend and extend feet and legs even under
slight resistance on my part. The power of eversion and inversion was returning. She could walk without assistance,
and with a much steadier and less waddling gait. No regurgitation of food had occurred since she came under my
treatment.

July 16th. The patient had again been treated four times.
On the 14th she walked a considerable part of the way to the
clinic without help, and also walked up three flights of stairs,
whereas previously she had to be carried up. Her voice had
lost the nasal accent, and the general appearance was greatly
improved.

July 23d. Treated three times since last report. During
the last few days she had experienced some pain in the ankles
and knees, because she had passed a good deal of time out of
doors. She had also felt a prickling sensation in the throat
toward the ears. By the above date these symptoms had disappeared. She could turn round without staggering, and
walked well.

August 2d. The patient was treated three times during
the preceding week, and on this occasion she had walked unassisted from her home to the clinic, and back again—in all

about an English mile and a quarter. She had regained her strength, and made all the movements well. Those at the ankle and knee-joint were executed with considerable force. She could stand quite steady with her eyes closed. She both looked and felt perfectly well, and could now be considered restored to health.

The patient had no treatment during the week following the 2d August, as I was away from Leipsic. She came again and was treated on the 9th, the 12th, and for the last time on the 16th, when she was dismissed as cured.

The patellar reflex had not returned, but, according to Dr. Moebius's experience, this generally does not appear until some time after the restoration of the muscular power.

On each occasion the patient was treated from half an hour to three-quarters of an hour.

From advices which I received up to the end of 1887, I was glad to learn that the patient continued in perfect health.

Treatment.—Each day of treatment I gave her the shakings for the throat (Figs. 20–23) with frictions over the facial nerve; pétrissage of the legs and gluteal region, and tapotement of the back—both accompanied by nerve frictions; and succeeding that other passive and then active movements, as seen in Figs. 55, 57, 68, etc.

In order to remove the waddling walk, I gave the movement shown in Fig. 71.

VII. NEURALGIA IN THE RIGHT FRONTAL REGION.

Gendarme-Sergeant Stanislaus R., 31 years of age, entered the Marine Hospital, Pola, on the 11th of December, 1888.

A year before, the patient had malaria, which left behind an intermittent neuralgia. He now complained of severe pain in the right frontal region, which had continued for several days.

He was treated for about ten minutes, when the pain disappeared.

Progress.—December 12th. Yesterday afternoon he felt slight pain for about an hour.

December 13th. Had no pain the day before.

Up to the 17th felt quite well. On that day he was dismissed as cured.

Treatment.—Frictions over the supraorbital nerve, and over the second cervical pair of nerves, produced sharp pain exactly at the place in the head where the patient suffered most. These nerves were treated—the first one with vibrations in the centripetal direction, the latter pair with light frictions and constant pressure. The patient was subjected to this treatment for ten minutes every morning.

VIII. Sciatica.

Joseph Scopac, sailor, 23 years old, contracted a gonorrhœa on the 18th of June, 1888. On the 5th of July cystitis set in; on the 2d August, pain in the left gluteal region; on the 28th August, conjunctivitis (left eye); 29th August, ciliary injection; 31st August, œdema palpebrarum; 1st September, iritis with bleeding into the anterior chamber and dimness of the cornea; 5th September, intra-ocular pressure decreased; 8th September, pain in left leg; 20th September, in left ankle; 5th October, pain in the neck.

The patient says that when the pain in the eyes increases, it also gets worse in the leg; 15th October, the ciliary injection decreased; 22d October, the glands in the neck and groin were swollen, and there were white patches on the tonsils. For these, mercurial ointment and iodide of potash were prescribed.

On December 6th the patient complained of pains in the left hip-joint, and especially in the middle, between the trochanter major and the tuber ischii; muscular weakness which caused waddling toward left side when walking. Lying on the right side, he could not lift the left leg in the least without help.

On the left eye there was immobility of the pupil; dimness of the lens; the fingers could scarcely be counted at a distance of 2 metres; small ciliary injection on the lateral edge of the cornea.

On the right eye the papilla and surrounding parts were red, and could hardly be distinguished from each other. No pains; sight good.

The treatment was started on the 6th December.

Progress.—December 10th. No pain, only weakness in the leg, which makes the walk difficult. Ciliary injection gone.

December 14th. Walks straighter.

December 17th. Walks well, looks much better, can make nearly as much resistance with the affected leg as with the sound one.

December 18th. Discharged as cured from the sciatica.

Treatment.—The patient lay in the prone position. Transverse frictions were for some minutes made over the great sciatic nerve where it passes between the great trochanter and the tuber ischii. The nerve was followed in its course as far down as the popliteal space, and frictions were also given over the sensory branches coming out through the posterior sacral foramina.

For the muscular weakness I employed pétrissage and the other passive and active movements shown in Figs. 69–71.

For the eyes, I gave vibrations over them; frictions and vibrations on the sensory branches of the fifth nerve coming out round the orbit; and lastly, frictions on the eye itself (Figs. 33, 39).

IX. SCIATICA.

J. Slobec, foreman at the Pola Naval Arsenal, 47 years old, caught a severe cold on the 5th February, 1889. He was obliged to take to his bed for pain in his left leg, and remained under treatment at home for a fortnight. Then he was transferred to the hospital, and on the 22d of the same month he came under my care.

The patient was very tall, looked haggard and thin, and the cheeks were sunken in. He suffered from intense pain in the left leg. It started from the gluteal region, and went right down to the heel and the sole of the foot.

The pain continued constantly through day and night. He was unable to obtain sleep.

He could not stand on his left foot, but kept it forward, touching the ground only with the toes; and he held the knee bent, the gluteal region drawn in.

Neither could he draw himself up to his usual height. The pain grew worse on standing. He could only walk with the greatest difficulty from the ward to the operation room, and then he needed a stick in one hand, and an ambulance man to steady him up on the other side. He took very small steps.

8

The skin peeled off in large flakes over the gluteal region, caused by strong applications of iodine tincture. Frictions over the great sciatic nerve in the gluteal region and all down its course cause a most severe pain.

The left gluteal region was sunken in; the muscles were loose and relaxed.

Progress.—I treated him at once—in the morning. The pain was greatly diminished after I had continued for eighteen minutes.

February 23d. The previous day he was nearly free from pain until six o'clock in the evening, but it did not then, or in the night, get nearly so intense as formerly, and therefore he slept some hours. He found walking a little easier.

February 24th, 25th. Not treated.

February 26th. The improvement on the 23d had continued.

February 27th. Had felt very much better during yesterday, and slept well during the night. After the treatment he walked away unassisted, and held himself fairly straight. He used the left leg well.

March 1st. He does not feel any pain during the day, if he keeps quiet; when he walks, he feels some in the gluteal region. Walks with a long step. He feels a little weak at the hip-joint, and therefore he does not trust himself to walk much; holds himself more erect; can stand about for a long time without experiencing pain; sleeps as soundly as when he was completely well.

March 4th. Yesterday he walked for twenty minutes in the forenoon, and twenty in the evening, in one stretch, without feeling any pain.

March 6th. He can walk without a stick, and with a long stride. Walked for about an hour.

March 7th. Started active movements.

March 9th. Had the day before gone down one flight of stairs, and walked for an hour in the forenoon and one in the afternoon; had subsequently felt a little pain in the evening, but it soon passed away. When he walks up-stairs, he feels rather weak in the gluteal muscles on the left side.

March 11th. Previous day walked about a good deal; also down two flights of stairs and up again. He still felt the weakness in the gluteal region, but the pain did not return.

March 18th. On Saturday he had paid a visit to his own house, where he remained over Sunday. He felt well all the time. Has only a kind of prickling in the calf, after walking for some hours. The weakness in the gluteal region is now so unimportant as to cause scarcely any trouble at all.

March 19th. Walked about in town for six hours yesterday; part of the time up hill; no bad consequences; slept well; felt no weakness in the gluteal region. The muscles have regained their firmness and tone.

March 22d. Walked six hours on the 20th, seven hours on the 21st, on both occasions partly in rain, without any bad results.

March 23d. Caught cold again, when the left leg was seized with trembling, and he felt slight pain in the gluteal region and the popliteal space. This quickly passed away when he had rested a little, and this morning he was as well as ever.

March 28th. Has had no treatment since the 23d. Has every day walked from seven to nine hours, and felt well all the time. The branch of the arsenal with which he is connected is the waterwork department, and this necessitates much walking, as his workmen are posted not only in different parts of the building, but also in the town as well. This day I treated him for the last time. I met him since in the town, and he told me he felt well. One day he had even had to walk eleven hours.

Treatment.—As I had observed the great effect produced in cases of traumatic and rheumatic lumbago by vibrations over the most painful places, I decided to adopt this form of treatment here, and to try it on its own merits. In the first of the two cases of sciatica mentioned above, and previously, I had always used frictions, but they give more pain at the time of application. This man suffered so frightfully, that I would not have recourse to them, unless they were absolutely necessary.

The patient was placed in the prone position, with the left leg crossed over the right one, as in Fig. 5. I then placed the last phalanx of my thumb (the linen intervening between it and the skin) over the great sciatic nerve just where it comes out of the pelvis (Fig. 72), and gave vibrations, during the first day for eighteen minutes, and on the following days for fifteen minutes. The good effect of this procedure was quickly manifest. Treated once a day. The active movements which I gave are shown in Figs. 57, 58, 69.

The patient had no treatment on February 24th and 25th,

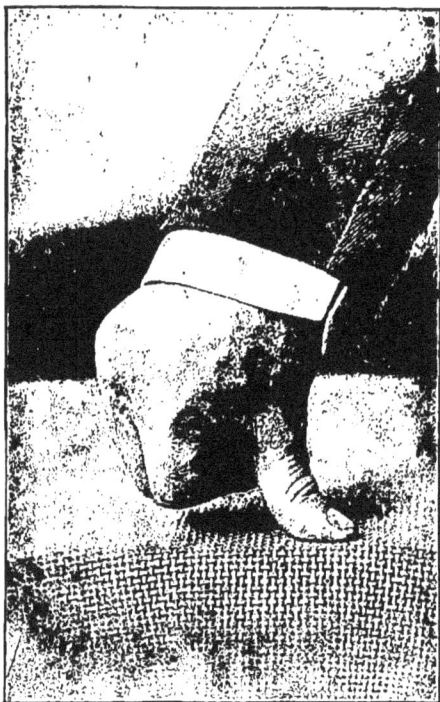

Fig. 72.

March 3d, 16th, 17th, 24th, 25th, 26th, 27th. He was thus treated only twenty-six times before the above result was obtained.

X. Traumatic Lumbago and Sciatica in the Right Leg.

Mr. E., 38 years of age, met with an accident in May, 1887. His horse shied just as he was in the act of mounting. The stirrup strap broke, and he was very nearly thrown off. At the moment he felt some pain in the lower part of his back, and this grew worse during the next three or four days. It gradually extended down the legs, especially the right one. He had also a feeling of heat inside the pelvis. He was treated for about five weeks with massage in Gothenburg, and he gradually grew better. During the illness he continued riding on horseback for several hours each day. In October, 1887, while making a sudden pull to get on a riding boot, the same pain again set in. This time the pain was at its height in about four to five hours. He was again treated with massage in Gothenburg for two months, until he got quite well.

Present History.—On the 8th of February, 1888, he lifted a very heavy weight. He felt some little pain in the lumbar region at the same place as before, and this increased until Tuesday, the 14th, when the patient had great difficulty in walking, moving the back, or standing. When he had been in any one position for a little time (*e.g.*, standing, sitting, or lying) he could only change it with the greatest difficulty and pain.

The right leg could not be stretched properly at the knee-joint. The neuralgia in the ischias was of a sharp shooting nature, and felt most in the gluteal region between the great trochanter and the tuber ischii, in the popliteal space, and the back of the leg, somewhat to its inner side. There was also a feeling of cold radiating from each side of the coccyx over the gluteal regions. The sensory nerves over the sacrum were very sensitive to pressure and friction.

Progress.—On Tuesday, the 14th, I began the treatment. The pain was relieved after the manipulation, as also on the following day; but at night he caught a severe cold, and the pain was greater than ever.

February 15th, 16th, 17th. Treated twice on each of these days. On the last he was sufficiently recovered to be out all the evening.

February 26th. The pain in the back had nearly disappeared. In the ischias and other branches of the sacral nerves plexus, the pain still returned after long walks.

March 3d. The stiffness in the leg nearly gone. Can walk without difficulty and pain.

March 10th. Not treated on the 4th, 5th, and 6th, as he had been travelling about sightseeing, which means much walking; but still he felt well all the time. The treatment was continued for another week.

Treatment.—Frictions over the ischias and sacral sensory branches, pétrissage over the lumbar region, and vibrations over the more sensitive places. Active movements from the very first day, as in Figs. 56, 71.

The exercise shown in Fig. 56 had to be begun at the floor with the toes steadied against the wall, and when the treatment finished it was made at normal height, with the heel as high up as the buttock.

XI. Rheumatic Lumbago.

F., 32 years old, Captain in the Imperial Austrian Navy, caught cold after a steam bath, on the 15th December, 1888. On the 17th he came up to the Marine Hospital.

He complained of pain in the whole lumbar region, radiating down over the gluteal regions. On examination it was found that the pain was greatest on a level with the transverse processes of the fourth lumbar vertebra. He could not undress unaided, could not walk straight, and could not bend the back. He had for over a year suffered more or less from rheumatism.

Progress.—After the first treatment the patient could move freely, and the pain ceased.

December 18th. Yesterday, toward evening, the pain came back, but was not so violent as before. After the treatment to-day it again ceased.

December 19th. The pain did not reappear. Could jump over the operation table after the treatment.

December 20th, 21st, 22d. The back was completely free from pain; all movements easy. Treatment stopped.

On the 21st, the patient complained of pain over the metatarso-phalangeal joint of the little toe. There was a dark red swelling, one inch long and half an inch broad, which was very tender to the touch. During the last few days we had had very cold weather, which had occasioned this frost-bite. After the treatment, which consisted of pétrissage and vibrations, the pain and the tension were greatly diminished.

December 22d. No tension; pain only on strong pressure.

The patient was treated for about a quarter of an hour once a day. The frost-bite was manipulated for a few minutes.

XII. Traumatic and Rheumatic Lumbago.

Dèlise, 42 years old, working man at the Naval Arsenal, Pola, came under my treatment on the 10th of February, 1889.

The patient had, during the month of May, 1888, lifted a heavy piece of iron, and had broken down under the weight. He then felt some pain in the lumbar region of the back. He continued working, although the pain gradually grew worse. He also caught cold, and this, too, settled in his back. He was in a very short time unfit for heavy labor, and only light work was given him.

After a few weeks, in the month of June, he could not go on with this either, because of the severe pain in his back, not only on moving it, but also when quiet. He was treated by several physicians in private practice, both at Pola and Trieste, but none of them could give him relief. In October, 1888, he entered the Marine Hospital, and after some weeks got rather better, when he left. Soon the pains set in again with their former intensity, and they became so severe that he was unable to obtain any sleep during the night, and entirely lost his appetite. He re-entered the hospital, and I was asked to treat him.

On the 10th of February his condition was as follows:

The patient looked very pale and worn, the cheeks were deeply sunken, and he had a very distressed expression of countenance. He complained of severe and constant pain in the lumbar region, radiating down over the gluteal regions; it was worse at night, and he got very little rest. Sometimes the agony was so great that he screamed out loudly.

He could not stand for more than a minute or two at a time, and then bent forward. He was incapable of dressing or undressing without help.

When he was lying on the operation table, face downward, the upper part of the lumbar region, at the first and second vertebræ, had not the normal curve, but was slightly bent backward. Opposite here the pain was most intense to friction or pressure. In this locality, also, the patient said he felt the pain greatest without being touched. He was extremely sensitive on the sides on the way down to the base of the spine. The great sciatic nerves responded painfully to friction.

Progress.—February 10th. I treated him at once. As the illness had lasted so long, I kept on for twenty-five to thirty minutes. The pain was then considerably diminished. The reaction ensued, and he became very weak, as if tired out, and he could not stand. He had to be carried down.

February 11th. During the previous day the patient had felt a great deal better, and had enjoyed more rest than for several months back, his sleep being less disturbed and the pain much easier. When it set in during the night, he tried himself to imitate my manipulation, and obtained relief by it. When he left the room, the other doctors present called my attention to his conspicuously free walk.

February 12th. He had slept through the whole night. The radiating pain over the gluteal region had gone, and only the original places in the lumbar region were painful. The patient looked brighter, and laid himself down on the operating table without any difficulty.

February 13th. Slept well; pain absent except on moving. During the night he felt only a kind of tenderness in the back.

February 16th. Slept well; entirely free from pain during the night. He has a keen appetite, which he has not had for many months.

February 18th. Feels pain only on quick movements. Began free active movements. Peculiarity in back gone.

February 26th. Has dressed unaided. Can, with arms extended upward, bend sideways and forward without any assistance. The pain produced by pressure or frictions greatly diminished. He can walk about for a considerable time without getting worse.

March 5th. Has for several days been free from pain after walking; he is about nearly the whole day; makes the active movements better and better each morning.

March 9th. He was so much improved that he could be sent from the hospital, but was to continue the treatment for some days yet. The active movements go very well. Bending forward he can touch the floor with his hands. In the morning these movements hurt him slightly at the beginning, but in the afternoon he feels nothing.

March 16th. Treatment stopped. He has to continue the active movements at home. After a week he resumed work at the arsenal.

Treatment.—In rheumatic and traumatic lumbago I always confine my treatment to the places which I find to be most painful to frictions. So I did in these two cases.

I placed my hands as shown in Fig. 73, the first phalanx of the thumb on one side of the spine, and those of the fore and long fingers on the other, over those situations which gave most pain. (It should be noted that the actual tips of the fingers are not applied.) Then I gave light vibrations and

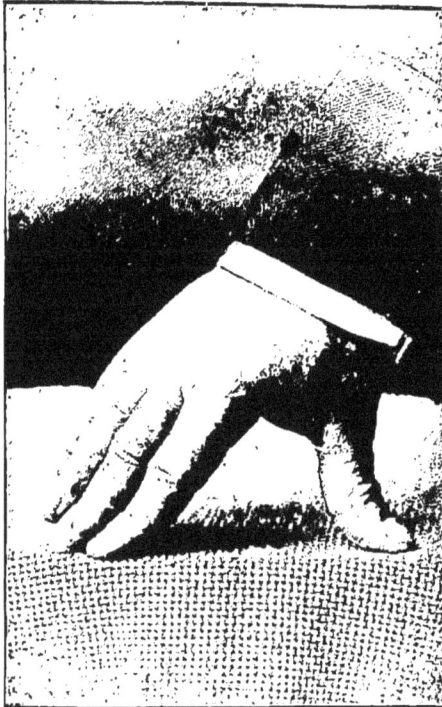

FIG. 73.

frictions alternately, and following these in both cases free active movements, consisting simply in bending, and turning in different directions, due attention being paid to correct positions.

At first, when these active exercises are made, I always give pétrissage at the seat of the pain, while the patient is moving. This eases it, and the movement goes better.

In the second case the patient was treated once in the

morning for twenty minutes, with the exception of the first day. After he had begun the active exercises, he repeated them once every afternoon.

XIII. STIFF NECK.

H. E., working man at the Naval Arsenal, 48 years of age, entered the Marine Hospital, Pola, on the 15th November, 1888.

Three months previously he had had a fever, after which stiffness of the neck and severe headache remained, the latter in the occipital region. The stiffness and the headache gradually increased. The headache was somewhat eased by the patient lying down on his back. At the infirmary he was treated with antipyrine and salicylate of soda. Of the first he had altogether taken about 9 grammes, of the latter 40 grammes.

On the 10th of December, 1888, he came under my care. His head was then immovable in all directions; the occipital headache was very marked; the cervical muscles were tender down to the shoulders. Sometimes the pain even passed down the arms. The slightest friction over the great occipital nerves gave intense pain.

Progress.—On the above date I started the treatment. The patient could move his head pretty well sideways and forward and backward after the first sitting.

December 11th. The improvement of the day before continued. After the treatment the pain was greatly diminished, and the movements were freer.

December 14th. Treatment and the movements, which are now normal in all directions, are painless. No headache.

December 15th. No treatment.

December 16th. Complained of noise in the ears and pain in front of them, tenderness of the sterno-mastoid, and tenderness and crackling in the temporo-maxillary joint.

December 17th. Noise in the ear lessened, as also the pain in the sterno-mastoid muscle, the pain in front of the ear, and crackling in the joint.

December 18th. Noise in the ear nearly gone. No pain anywhere.

December 19th. Discharged as cured.

Treatment.—The greatest pain was found at the places of attachment of the muscles of the neck to the occipital bone. There, then, I principally applied the treatment, which consisted in pétrissage. The muscles themselves I treated only very slightly.

On the pétrissage followed passive and active movements, as in Figs 47, 48, 62.

Here it was seen that a muscle acting under resistance contracts more forcibly—*i.e.*, the range of movement is greater —than when it does so unimpeded.

Lastly, I made light vibrations over the occipital nerves.

The noise in the ears, the pain in front of them, and the crackling in the joint, were treated with pétrissage and frictions over the facial and anterior auricular nerves.

XIV. Tendo-vaginitis.

K. K., sailor, 22 years old, came under treatment on the 12th of December, 1888. Six days previously inflammation had set in in the tendons of the extensores primi internodii and

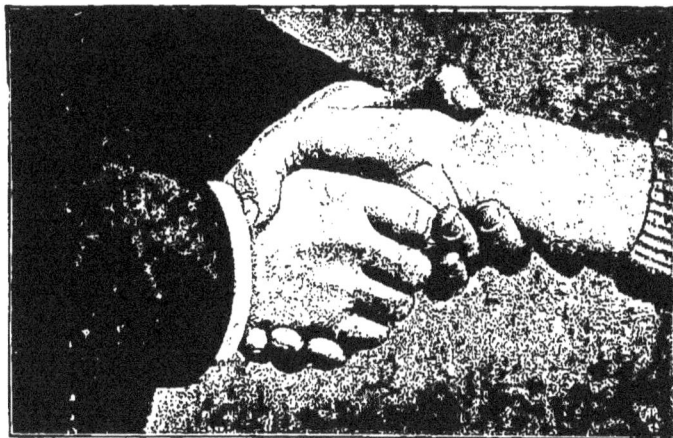

Fig. 74.

ossis metacarpi pollicis. It began spontaneously. The tendons were thickened for about 5 cm. in length, where they lie in their sheath of the annular ligament; strong friction sounds on movement; pain on touch and movement.

December 14th. Friction sounds still present, but only in

the neighborhood of the joint, absent higher up; pain is only felt in the morning.

December 17th. Friction sounds can nowhere be heard. Movement also in the morning completely painless.

December 18th. Dismissed cured.

Treatment.—I gave at first pétrissage; afterward passive movements, with strong extension of the affected tendons; these were followed by active movements under resistance for the affected muscles.

While I gave the pétrissage I bent the patient's hand strongly toward the ulnar side in order to keep the tendons extended, and thus prevent them from moving (Fig. 74).

The patient was treated every day from eight to ten minutes.

XV. Wound of the Cornea.

Miss M., dressmaker, Clapham, injured her eye on the 12th of December, 1887. She was shaking a towel when with one of the corners she struck her right eye sharply. Pain set in, and grew worse during the night. It was so severe as to prevent her from sleeping.

On the morning of the 13th she went to a doctor, who told her there was a cut "over the dark part of the eye." He put two drops of "something" into the eye, and gave her a lotion to bathe it with. I called in the evening to treat the lady of the house where she was working. As the pain had steadily increased during the day, I was asked to look at her eye, and if possible relieve her.

When I saw her about 9:30 P.M., the eyelids were swollen and red, the conjunctiva injected, the vessels in the sclerotic part of it enlarged and shooting toward the cornea. On examining the cornea, I found a wound close over the horizontal diameter, and a little to the outer side of the pupil. The wound did not now present the appearance of a cut, but had spread on all sides, and was somewhat larger than an ordinary pin's head. The edges were irregular and seemed turned up. There was a slight discharge of pus, much lachrymation and photophobia; the pupil was very dilated and fixed; it was not round but uneven. All the branches of the fifth nerve responded very painfully to friction.

Progress and Treatment.—I gave vibrations on the eye,

and frictions over the branches of the fifth nerve. I had to pursue the treatment for about twenty to twenty-five minutes before the pain entirely disappeared. As the lotion had done no good, I told her to discontinue it, to keep the eye covered, and to abstain from work.

December 14th. The pain came back later on, during the night, but only very slightly. She slept fairly well. The swelling and redness of the eyelids were greatly reduced; the injection of the conjunctiva, both on lids and eye, was also considerably diminished. The pupil reacts only slightly and sluggishly. On looking at a strong gaslight only little pain is felt.

December 15th. Pain in the eye completely gone. None during the night. Upper lid nearly normal; injection of eye less than on preceding day; pupil reacts better; wound in cornea healed up.

December 16th. No lachrymation; eye clear; can read ordinary newspaper print.

After a week's treatment she was able to do needle-work without difficulty or pain.

Treatment during all days, excepting the first, lasted ten minutes in the forenoon, five minutes in the evening. On the 15th I also gave nerve vibrations on the eye itself (Fig. 40). The treatment was continued for some days longer, and was given only in the evening for a few minutes.

XVI. Scar on Palmar Surface of Right Hand.

Lieutenant P., of the Fort Artillery Battalion at Pola, consulted me on the 14th December, 1888. Four weeks previously he had cut his hand through falling with a spirit-lamp. The scar began about 1 cm. below the right wrist, and passed in half-moon shape over the anti-thenar until near the ulnar edge of the hand. It was about 6 cm. long, immovable, retracted, edges hardened and elevated. When the ring finger was stretched it was considerably drawn in at the wrist. The hand and the forearm were weak, so that the patient could not use them. The feeling in the little finger and ulnar side of ring finger was much diminished; friction over the ulnar nerve causing no reaction in these places. Adduction of the little finger not possible.

The first treatment was given on the 14th December, and after it the feeling in the little finger began to return.

December 15th. More power in the hand.

December 16th. Scar not retracted so much; edges softer.

December 17th. If the hand is placed flat on the table, the patient can adduct the little finger. Scar less depressed, and the drawing in at the wrist, on stretching the ring finger, is hardly perceptible. Scar in the hand freely movable.

December 18th. At the wrist it is free from parts under-

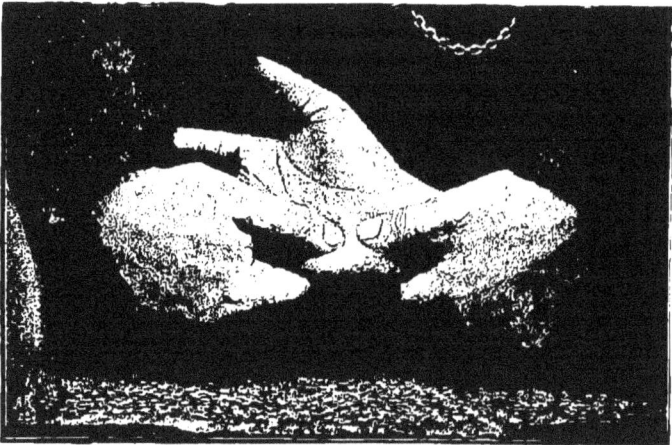

FIG. 75.

neath for about ¾ cm. The feeling in the ring and little fingers greatly improved. Power in the arm and hand normal.

Treatment.—I gave pétrissage over the elevated and hardened surroundings of the scar. In order to detach it from the parts underneath, the two thumbs were placed opposite each other, with the volar surface of the ungual phalanx on the scar, at a distance of about 1 cm., and in the direction of it. The thumbs were then moved toward each other (Fig. 75). Of course care was taken that the parts of the scar underneath the thumbs moved with them. In this way the adhesions were mechanically torn down.

The weakness in the little finger was caused partly by direct injury of the muscles, and partly by impaired power of the ulnar nerve. That the nerve was actually affected was manifest from the direction of the scar, and from the fact that it did not respond to frictions over its course.

The weakness of the muscles was treated with pétrissage and active movements under resistance. For the diminution of feeling I gave frictions over the ulnar nerve.

XVII. Severe Bruise of the Face and Concussion of the Brain, in Consequence of a Fall from a Dog-cart.

Mrs. A. A. C., about 50 years of age, residing at Kensington, London, met with an accident on the 7th August, 1888. The dog-cart in which she was driving came in collision with a heavily-laden van, and she was thrown out. She fell on her face, was stunned by the blow, and taken to St. Thomas's Hospital, where restorative measures were applied. Gradually she regained consciousness, and her daughter, who accompanied her, then brought her to me. She felt very giddy while driving over. She had fallen on the left side of the face. The chin received the hardest blow, and was very badly bruised and open. The lower lip was cut through by the teeth in two places. The greatest swellings were over the two named places, and over the malar bone. The nose was swollen, but not broken. The right maxillary joint was very tender, and she could only open the mouth very little. Considerable pain was present in this region. The head ached.

Progress and Treatment.—The pain was taken away and the swelling greatly diminished by vibrations and light kneadings. The wounds through the lip were brought together with silk plaster, as she would not allow me to stitch them up; that on the chin was left open. I also gave nerve frictions in the neck for the headache. The patient felt well enough on leaving.

August 8th. When she called at my house the following morning, there was no dark discoloration anywhere, except on the lower lid of the eye. The lower jaw was more movable. She had slept pretty well, but was now and then awakened if she turned over to the side on which the injuries were. All the sensory branches on the skull and forehead were exceedingly sensitive.

I went to her house in the evening and treated her again. Treatment same as yesterday. In the afternoon a feeling of sickness with giddiness and severe headache set in, and increased until seven o'clock, when I paid my visit. She could not bear any light in the room; would on no account open her eyes. The pulse was seventy beats a minute, lightly irregular. The seat of the pain she said was deep in the middle of the head. She was somewhat drowsy. I made frictions over the second pair of cervical nerves and light vibrations on the eyes (Fig. 32)—in all for about twenty minutes. The headache was relieved by this, and she could open the eyes, the gaslight causing her no inconvenience.

The feeling of sickness remained, and for it I gave general pétrissage of the abdomen, accompanied by light vibrations in the pit of the stomach. The sickness then passed away. She fell asleep during the latter part of the treatment, but awoke in an hour with the same sensation of nausea, which was again taken away, and she again slept. This happened three times successively up till midnight, when I went away. I remained so long because it was the first case of that kind I had subjected to this treatment.

August 9th. After I left last night the patient had slept off and on until the morning. The headache was gone and also the sickness, but she said she did not feel quite clear in her head. There was some yellowness about the bruised places, all of which healed very well. The scab over the bruise on the chin peeled off. The branches of the fifth nerve on the forehead were still very tender. Frictions over them caused a slight feeling of sickness.

Treated once in the forenoon.

August 10th. Yesterday afternoon the sickness returned, but only in a very modified form, and she had also a slight headache; both soon passed away. Slept very well during the night. No feeling of sickness or headache this morning. Head clear. All bruises and cuts healed up.

August 11th. The patient felt very well. I stopped the treatment, but told her to let me know at once if sickness or headache reappeared. They did not.

XVIII. Ulcerated External Hemorrhoids.

Mr. C. S., 42 years of age, civil engineer, London. The patient has a nervous temperament. He leads a generous life, and is very plethoric. Digestion disordered for several months

back; has for a long time had a nervous cough, probably reflex from the stomach. At the beginning of January, 1888, he
went down to Brighton for change of air, as he felt considerably out of sorts. While there, he read of the wonderful prop-
erties of certain pills, and their purifying effect on the blood.
He at once proceeded to try them, and in rather large doses.
The consequence was a violent diarrhœa, followed by an
equally obstinate constipation, with the diagreeable sequel of
external piles. He now went from Brighton to Hastings,
where he became worse, and had to lie in bed. The piles gradually began to inflame and ulcerate. At last, Mr. S. was advised to return to London, in order to undergo an operation.
The idea of this rather terrified him, and he came first to me
on the 21st of February, 1888.

There were no less than seven ulcers clustering all round
the anus, and the surrounding redness, which was very intense, extended high up on the gluteal regions. Several of the
ulcers were three-quarters of an inch long and a quarter of an
inch broad. The edges were elevated.

I wished to make complete internal examination, but the
patient would not allow it, because of the pain it caused him
at Hastings. He suffered greatly on walking. The stools
gave him much pain, and this remained for a considerable
time afterward.

Progress.—I treated him at once for rather more than half
an hour, when I succeeded in relieving the pain and irritation.
In the evening I occupied the same length of time.

February 22d. He felt considerably easier, and the redness
on the gluteal regions had disappeared.

February 24th. He had improved from day to day, and
could now walk about comfortably.

February 26th. The ulcers had entirely lost their inflammatory appearance, had sunken, and were diminished; the
stools gave no pain.

February 27th. The patient started on a six weeks' travelling tour on the Continent, the ulcers soon healed, and he
had no discomfort whatever.

Treatment.—I first washed the ulcers with a solution of
corrosive sublimate (1 : 2,000). Then I placed a moist piece of
lint over the particular ulcers to be treated. Over this again
I laid gutta-percha, in order to prevent the heat of my hands

9

being transmitted to the inflamed piles when I made the vibrations. I subjected one side at a time to manipulation. I treated the patient twice a day up to the 24th, the duration of the treatment decreasing with each sitting. I also gave frictions over the sensory nerves on the sacrum, and over those on the gluteal region. After that I made shakings and tapotement of the liver; nerve frictions in the back opposite the lower angle of the scapula on the right side; and lastly, general pétrissage of the abdomen. I supplied the patient with some corrosive sublimate solution and lint for the journey, in order to keep the ulcers clean.

XIX. Stiff Knee Forcibly Broken Down.

The following case dates as far back as the summer of 1884, when I was in charge of my brother's institution in London. Dr. Thomas Easton, of Stranraer, was also there studying the treatment. He has been kind enough to send me the notes which he took of the case at the time. They are as follows:

Paul W., Holly Bank, Sheffield, engineer, suffered from rheumatism for many years. It was first contracted at a colliery work, where he was often exposed to damp and cold. At first the rheumatism was mostly confined to his right shoulder. In February, 1883, he felt the pain in his right knee, but after applying cold water to it for a day or two it disappeared. He had then a period of six months during which his health was very good. In November of the same year the rheumatism returned, and his right shoulder was severely affected. At this time he had a fall, bruising the right knee. The rheumatism spread more over the body, attacking the left hand, and finally seemed to settle permanently in the right knee. The patient was then confined to bed for ten weeks, during which his knee was kept at rest.

Hot fomentations and blistering were tried, and subsequently mercurial ointment, but the result of the illness was a stiff knee. A month or two later, the patient put himself under the care of Mr. Kellgren, of Eaton Square. He remained one month under his treatment, but only made slight progress. Mr. Wood then went to Cardiff, and his medical advisers there partially broke down his knee in two separate operations under chloroform and ether. After the operations the knee was put up in a bent splint.

In the autumn of 1884 the patient returned to Eaton Square, and, in the absence of Mr. Kellgren, the treatment which he had before received was recommenced by Mr. Arvid Kellgren. He made but slow progress, and suffered great pain. It was then suggested to him that the knee might be more forcibly broken down under chloroform. I accordingly put him deeply under chloroform, while Mr. Arvid Kellgren broke down the adhesions round the knee. The operation was performed twice, at an interval of a fortnight. The first breaking down was only partial, but on the second occasion, on the 10th of September, the knee adhesions were completely broken down, the leg being flexed on the thigh as much as it can be under normal conditions. The pain after the operation was very severe, and the swelling around the joint considerable, but after pétrissage and effleurage had been applied, the pain almost disappeared.

Thursday, September 11th. The patient passed a tolerably good night, though he was rather feverish. The pain only gave slight discomfort. Spasmodic jerks were felt during the night at the knee-joint.

On examination, the joint was found to be more swollen than on the previous evening, and there was slight discoloration in front, just below the patella. The joint was then moved, active and passive movements being tried. After the movements pétrissage was given. Pulse, 82; temperature, 99°. The patient expressed himself much relieved after treatment.

Friday, September 12th. The patient felt feverish. Temperature, 99.5°; pulse, 84. The tension in the knee was greater, and the area of discoloration had extended much further in front. Movements and massage were again applied. The same evening his temperature rose to 100°, but after the treatment it fell to 99°.

Saturday, September 14th. Temperature, 99.2°; fell to 98.8° after treatment; pulse, 78. Swelling still great. The discoloration more diffused; pain less, but jerking spasms.

The same evening the temperature was 99.6°, and pulse 82. After treatment these were respectively reduced to 98.8° and 78. The swelling was still great, but the extravasation color was changed, and movement in the joint through a small limit was easier and without pain.

Monday, September 16th. Temperature, 99.2´; pulse, 84.
Swelling still considerable, and jerking pains annoying on
going off to sleep.

During the following days the pain on moving subsided in
a marked degree, and the discoloration and the swelling rapidly disappeared. On Sunday, the 15th, the patient had gone
down-stairs, and after a fortnight he came to Eaton Square.
On the 20th of October he left London, although we told him
that a longer stay was necessary. On the 1st November he
writes as follows: "I find I can walk fairly well, though the
leg does not bend much past the right angle, nor will it go
perfectly straight like the other."

As long as the patient stayed at home he was treated twice
a day, half an hour on each occasion; afterward once a day.

XX. Infra-clavicular Dislocation of the Left Humerus.

Marcus F., 47 years old, workingman, came to the Marine
Hospital at Pola on the 21st February, 1889, with the left
shoulder dislocated. He said that a cart-load of sand had
fallen upon him the day before. The pain in the left shoulder
was so great that he turned quite faint, and could not rise
without assistance. On examination of the shoulder, the head
of the humerus was found lying under the clavicle. The swelling from exudation was considerable, and extended over the
whole of the upper arm, on the inner side of which discoloration began to show itself.

On the 22d, in the morning, the patient was put under
chloroform, and the humerus replaced by circumduction. The
arm was afterward put in an ordinary sling.

February 23d. I began with passive movements—viz., pétrissage, effleurage, rolling (Fig. 50). Unnecessary movement
at the shoulder during the pétrissage and effleurage was prevented by stretching and adducting the arm to the side with
one hand, while I worked with the other.

February 24th. No treatment.

February 26th. The arm during the rolling could be carried as high up as the level of the shoulder. There was great
discoloration on the inner side of the upper arm. On the previous day the patient tried to move the arm himself, and had
got it partly dislocated again, the head of the humerus being

on the anterior and lower edge of the glenoid cavity. In order to prevent a recurrence of this, the arm was bandaged up over the chest. Began with active movements.

March 1st. He could stretch the arm horizontally forward, and if he steadied the hand against the wall of the room he could work it up until it reached nearly as high as the sound one. The rolling, extension, and flexion go much freer. When he half lies with the back steadied, I could without difficulty stretch his arm straight up. He could place his hand on his neck.

March 6th. The arm was left free, and he was told to move it about often during the day. He can reach as high up with the hand of the injured arm as with that of the sound one.

March 7th. The active movements under resistance show that the muscles round the affected shoulder have almost completely regained their strength. The topographical appearance of shoulder normal.

March 14th. Treated for the last time but allowed two days' rest from work.

The patient was treated once a day for about fifteen to twenty minutes, with the exception of the 24th and 25th February, and 3d and 10th of March, when no treatment was given.

XXI. Fracture of the Lower End of the Radius.

A. R., sailor, 20 years old, working in the engine-room. On the 10th of December, 1888, he fell on the dorsally flexed left hand. Severe pain, extravasation, and swelling ensued There was an oblique fracture of the lower end of the radius, starting at the ulnar side below, and going outward and upward. He had his arm in splints, which by my direction were removed, and they were not replaced so long as he remained under my care.

Progress and Treatment.—December 12th. I began the treatment, which consisted in pétrissage, effleurage, and other passive movements, rolling, etc. The patient felt considerably easier after the treatment, the pain at the fracture and joint being diminished.

December 15th. Swelling nearly gone. During the passive movements he feels some pain at the seat of fracture.

December 16th. He yet feels pain at the seat of the fracture from the passive movement. He can extend and flex the hand at the wrist nearly normally, and without any pain. As yet he cannot lift anything. The exudation has disappeared to such an extent that the flexor tendons are clearly seen. Active movements under light resistance have been started.

December 17th. During the night he had slept on the arm without any bad consequences. The active movements go better, yet he cannot lift anything; can close the hand completely and rather firmly. Free supination and pronation possible, but he feels pain at the seat of the fracture on resistance being made. The passive movements—such as rolling, flexion, and extension, etc.—are painless.

December 18th. Active flexion and extension movements can be made without the arm being steadied at the seat of the fracture.

December 21st. Stopped the treatment, as I left Pola. No movements gave pain—all were normal, and the patient could lift light articles, such as books, etc. The treatment lasted each day for about a quarter of an hour. When I gave pétrissage and effleurage, I steadied the whole arm on the table, and with the left hand I fixed the fractured place. During the other passive and active movements I grasped with one hand the fracture, so that thereby the pieces were kept from moving. As there was no one in Pola to continue this special form of treatment, the splints when I left were replaced.

XXII. STIFFNESS OF ELBOW-JOINT AFTER FRACTURE AT THE UPPER END OF THE RADIUS.

H. J., Lieutenant in the I. and R. Austrian Navy, came into the hospital at Pola on the 27th of January, 1889, having fallen on his right elbow from a bicycle. Great pain, immobility, and swelling were present at that joint.

January 28th. The contusion was strongly colored; abnormal movement and crepitation were felt about two fingers' breadth from the head of the radius. Plaster-of-Paris bandage was applied on the arm, which was held at a right angle and midway between supination and pronation.

February 18th. The plaster-of-Paris bandage was removed, and I was asked to correct the abnormal position.

There was very little mobility at the elbow. The amount of extension and flexion was about 20° in each direction, with the right angle taken as starting-point. Supination and pronation absent. The wrist-joint was stiff, and did not allow of much movement. It was also very weak.

He could only with the tip of his thumb touch the protruded chin, or the forehead when the head was bent forward. Could with difficulty pass the hand behind his back, and he was unable to move it higher than the lumbar region.

When the arm was passively extended, the tendon of the biceps muscle was felt to be very tense.

Swelling was still present, especially over the outer side of the elbow, and extended for some inches up and down, obscuring the contours. It pitted deeply on pressure, and remained so for some time.

Pain was felt on pressure over the swelling at the seat of fracture; at the elbow and wrist-joints on moving; and in the ulnar nerve, where it passes behind the internal condyle of the humerus, because round it exudation had settled and filled up the groove.

Treatment and Progress.—I took the case in hand on the 18th of February. The treatment consisted in pétrissage, effleurage, and other passive and active movements, some with, some without, resistance. I gave them all from the very first day. During the treatment, crackings were often heard from the tearing of organized exudations.

March 9th. The arm had regained its strength; the bending and stretching had so much improved that the angle formed during movement was 160°. Supination and pronation were already normal on the 6th; the patient could go through the fencing movements with the sword very well. No pain in the ulnar nerve on strong flexion; no movements caused pain, they were all performed with freedom and ease.

March 16th. The bending at the elbow was nearly normal; same with the stretching. Passing his hand behind his neck, the patient could touch between the shoulders with the fingers; and passing it behind the back, he could reach the shoulder of the same side (*i.e.*, the right one).

The patient had already, on the 9th, left the hospital to resume his naval duties. After the 16th he remained away for several days, and came afterward a few times for treatment.

The treatment lasted every day for about twenty minutes, and it continued a longer time than usual because of the short-

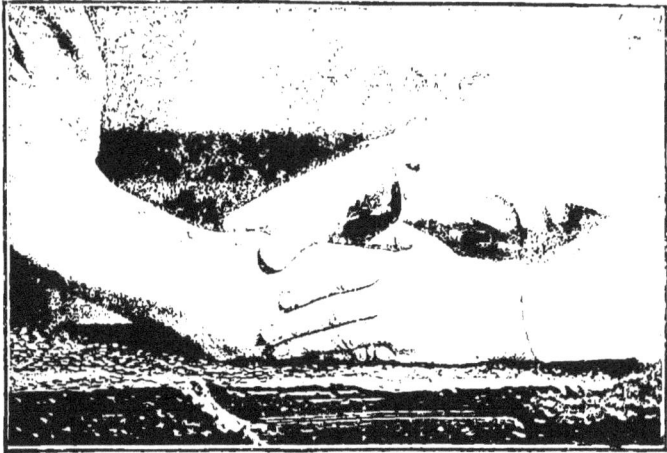

FIG. 76.

ening of the biceps muscles, and the pain in the ulnar nerve caused by the exudation round it.

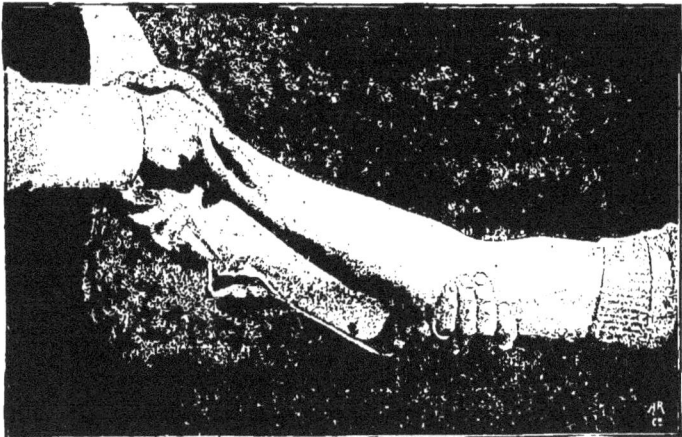

FIG. 77.

I should wish to draw attention to the following points in the accompanying illustrations of movements given during the treatment of the above case. In Fig. 76, showing pétrissage at the elbow over exudation there, it should be noticed how completely the position of the left hand steadies the arm.

I have treated fresh fractures round the elbow at once with pétrissage without causing the patient much pain, because steadiness of the arm was thus secured.

In Fig. 77 note the application of the hands for pronation and supination of the forearm. The one grasps the elbow, the other the hand, with two fingers passed down in front of the wrist.

In Fig. 78 we have the application of the hands for gradually breaking down a stiff wrist. Both hands are placed

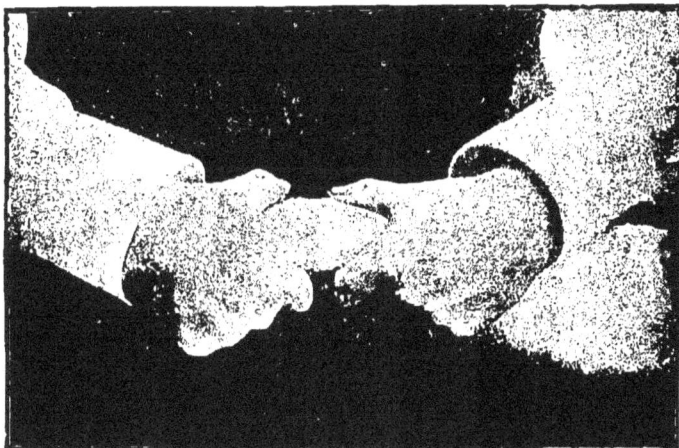

FIG. 78.

close to the joint. Passive extension and vibrations are made as we move it.

XXIII. DOUBLE FRACTURE OF FIBULA AT ITS LOWER THIRD, WITH FRACTURE OF THE EXTERNAL MALLEOLUS.

W. R., 24 years old, Lieutenant in the 97th Austrian Infantry Regiment, was carried to the Marine Hospital on the 1st of February, 1889. He had been riding on horseback. The horse fell, and he had his right foot under it. The foot was strongly inverted just after the accident. The patient complained of fearful pain, especially at the internal malleolus. The parts round the ankle were greatly swollen. Examination showed fracture of the fibula at its lower third, where crepitation was felt. The internal malleolus was also believed to be broken, but owing to the pain and excessive swelling it could not with certainty be decided to what extent. The leg was put in a Petit-boot. The pain grew so unendurable during the night that the patient had to send for the resident surgeon, who ordered an ice compress. On the 4th, several bullæ, each the size of a sixpence or more, made their appearance on the inner and lower part of leg and ankle. They contained serum; were opened and treated with iodoform bandage.

On the 12th of February I saw the patient for the first time. The foot and leg were immensely swollen, the swelling extending as high as the knee-joint. The exudation was rather firm, pitted everywhere deeply on pressure, and the pits remained long.

The skin had a greenish-yellow color. There were three especially painful places, and after the treatment had been given for some time the fractures could very well be made out. One was transverse 10 cm. high; another oblique, running from below upward and backward, and ending posteriorly about 3 cm. above the tip of the external malleolus. Both were on the fibula. On the internal malleolus there could be felt a longitudinal furrow, starting at the tip and going upward for a distance of 2 cm., and then bifurcating forward and backward, ending 4 cm. high anteriorly and 3 cm. posteriorly. It was thus easily to be seen that the injury had been caused by a crush. The bullæ were not completely healed. The foot was stiff.

Treatment and Progress.—It consisted as usual of pétrissage and effleurage; intermingled with and following on the former being other passive movements, such as rolling, extension, and flexion, etc.; then active movements, partly free, partly under resistance; and lastly, frictions over the internal and external popliteal nerves.

February 19th. The swelling has gone down on the leg, but remains round the ankle and upper part of the dorsum of the foot, although considerably diminished. The movements at the ankle go pretty well, and do not cause nearly so much pain as at first. The fractured pieces adhere well to each other. The bullæ have healed. They had delayed the treatment on the inner side of the ankle.

February 26th. The swelling round the ankle much diminished, and on the dorsum of the foot it is gone. The passive and active movements are scarcely felt at the fractures. The patient can move his feet freely. I decided to let him try to walk, which he did, steadied on both sides. He kept the foot still, both because he was somewhat nervous and because he felt pain in the joint when he rested his weight upon it. It was, he said, a sort of burning sensation. As I supposed that the pain was caused by exudation in the joint itself, I gave rolling of the foot, and passive extension and flexion, rather longer than usual. At the fractures he felt no movement on walking. The muscles of the calf are smaller on the injured leg, and do not act so well.

March 6th. Walked up and down the room for over five minutes. The foot turned very red, but there was no pain in the joint. He walks pretty quickly and steadily without assistance. He feels the foot somewhat stiff, from a dragging behind at the heel and internal malleolus. From to-day, the foot and leg lie free.

March 12th. He has walked more and more every day, and each time with greater ease. In order to diminish the stiffness and to stimulate the muscles of the calf, he had to make the movement shown in Fig. 58. When doing so for the first time, he slipped and twisted the foot again. This gave him pain at the seat of the fractures, but it speedily passed away on application of vibrations.

March 13th. During the night he had felt pain in all the fractured places, but it was very slight. Treated as usual and made to walk as before.

March 14th. Free from pain yesterday and last night. The swelling, which is very stubborn on the inner side of the ankle and round the Achilles tendon, has greatly subsided. The movements in the foot are normal, except dorsi-flexion, which is somewhat prevented by the Achilles tendon and by the tendons passing round the thickened internal malleolus. The muscular power developed is good. Is allowed to dress and go about the room; must, however, when sitting keep the leg in the horizontal position.

March 19th. Walked out yesterday morning for the first time. Had to go up and down two flights of stairs. Going down-stairs was somewhat difficult, but up-stairs not. Went

out again in the afternoon and walked about for an hour i
the hospital garden. The patient was not allowed to use hi
own boots, but used a pair of large ones.

March 23d.   Walked into town yesterday with his ordinar
boots on.   Felt nothing beyond a little stiffness in the ankle
He was on his feet for over three hours.   Walks with a ful
step.

March 30th.   Goes on leave next Monday, the 1st of Apri
Treated to-day for the last time.

The malleoli are thickend from the exudations at the seat
of the fractures.   They have the following measurements i

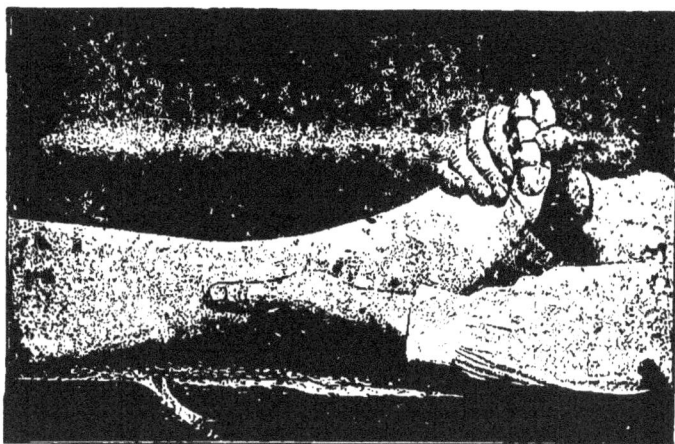

Fig. 79.

comparison to the sound ones: Internal malleolus on broker
side, $4\frac{1}{4}$ cm. broad; on sound side, $3\frac{1}{2}$ cm.   External malleolus
$3\frac{1}{2}$ cm. on broken side; 3 cm. on sound side.

The case ought to have been under manual treatment from
the very first day.   The exudation would then never have
been allowed to settle as it did, and the recovery would con
sequently have been very much quicker.

The illustration (Fig. 79) shows how the thumb is applied
alongside the fibula in order to act as a splint while we extend
and flex the foot.

I met the patient on my way to Vienna at the end o
April.   He then walked well, and it was only when he walked
very quickly that one could see that his foot had been injured

The patient had no treatment on the following dates: February 17th, 24th, and 25th, March 3d, 10th, 17th, 24th, 25th, 26th, and 27th.

Bearing in mind the structure of the foot, it will readily be seen that it is possible to evert and invert it without danger provided we take the precaution of placing the hand over the point of fracture, and the foot be held at a right angle to the leg. These movements do not, as we know, take place at the ankle-joint, but chiefly at the astragalus, scaphoid, and calcaneo-cuboid articulations.

XXIV. Double Fracture of the Fibula at its Lower Third.

On the 15th of January, 1887, Mrs. L., 43 years old, slipped and fell as she was stepping out of her carriage. She rose up and fell again. On both occasions she heard a distinct cracking in her left ankle. The second time of falling she fainted away.

On examination it was found that the fibula had sustained two fractures: one oblique, running from below forward and outward, about 10 cm. from the tip of the external malleolus; the other transverse about 3 cm. from the tip of the same malleolus. At the upper seat of injury the pieces of bone were somewhat displaced, and here the effusion appeared first; at the lower there was no displacement, but the fracture was felt very well when the foot was inverted.

Progress.—January 15th. Between the first two applications of the treatment on the day of the accident, the swelling did not increase very much, and the patient had no pain.

January 16th. During the preceding night, a considerable amount of effusion had collected round the ankle, over the dorsum of the foot, and upward as high as the upper third of the calf. It was not very tense, and pitted easily on pressure, but the depressions quickly disappeared. There was no discoloration. The patient had slept well and had had a painless night.

January 23d. The effusion has passed almost entirely away, remaining only over the fractures and on the inner side of the ankle; but the cause of its appearance in the latter place was, I believe, gout, which was present as a complication.

Over the whole of the leg in general no discoloration had been present, except a slight yellowish tinge; but high up on the posterior surface of the calf I noticed on the morning of the 17th a dark blue color, which indicated to me that I had not carried the treatment sufficiently far.

There has been no pain. The sleep had been undisturbed. The patient can extend and bend the foot to a considerable degree without much difficulty. Eversion and inversion slight. When the same active movements are made under resistance they go better.

January 30th. The effusion is gone, but it still remains over the fractures and inner side of ankle, although in a much smaller amount. All the movements can be performed easier and with more force.

February 6th. Scarcely any effusion over the fracture. On the inner side of the ankle it comes and goes, owing to the gouty condition. The patient has during the week walked about the room unassisted, simply steadying herself by the furniture. No movement perceptible at the seat of the fractures. Active movements performed with considerable force. Both they and the passive are nearly normal in range.

February 20th. The patient can walk quickly up and down stairs. The movements at ankle-joint normal in range and power. No abnormal thickening at the seats of the fractures.

Treatment.—No splints were applied. The deviation of the foot was corrected simply by muscular action. When the patient was sitting or lying, the foot was steadied at a right angle to the leg.

Pétrissage and effleurage were given from the very first, and also vibrations over the situation of the fractures. The former were administered for the effusion; the latter more especially for the pain. During the first days other passive movements, such as rolling, bending, stretching, eversion and inversion of the foot, were given in order to prevent exudation from organizing and causing stiffness. Active movements as in previous case.

The patient was not kept in bed a single day. She was helped down-stairs every morning, and had then to use the foot as little as she could at first, but it was always held at a right angle to the leg. From the third day, the patient was allowed to drive out, the same precaution being taken about the foot as when she was sitting in her room.

During the first weeks the treatment was given twice a day.

XXV. CYSTITIS.

Mr. L. R., 30 years of age, had for several months been troubled with a slight gleet. In order to get rid of it quickly, he had recourse to a 1-per-cent injection of nitrate of silver, which he had heard would produce an immediate cure. He used the injection so carelessly that a part of it passed into the bladder. This caused him extreme discomfort; so much so, that he was compelled to remain completely quiet for over an hour after its application.

It was a very warm summer day, and the patient in the afternoon took some ices. He very soon began to shiver, went home, and repaired to bed, where he was obliged to remain three days. Fever, vomiting, intense irritation of the bladder, pain in the perineum and lower part of the back and sacrum, set in. His appetite entirely left him, and he could only drink acidulated water, and take fluid food; there were constant calls to empty the bladder, which were accompanied and followed by intense irritation and a desire to void the urine though the bladder was empty. He had very little sleep at night.

On the fourth day, September 3d, 1888, when he came for treament, the above symptoms had slightly subsided. He looked worn and haggard, suffered from a feeling of great prostration, and bitterly repented having tried to work his own cure. He had no fever; the appetite had so far improved that he could take very light food. Walking was exceedingly disagreeable to him, as also driving, because both set up irritation in the bladder.

The urine deposited pus, mucus, triple phosphates of ammonia and magnesia.

Progress.—September 10th. The patient has been treated twice a day from the 3d. The very first treatment on that day gave him relief for some hours. He felt no discomfort on walking home. He passed a much better night, more rest and sleep being enjoyed. There has been a constant improvement from day to day. The urine is now passed two to three times a day, and he does not need to rise during the night. For the last two or three days he has had no feeling of irritation after emptying the bladder, but only a kind of weakness. The deposition of phosphates, mucus, and pus greatly diminished. The appetite is improving.

September 24th. The patient has been treated once a day since the last report. He caught cold on the 14th, and had a slight relapse, which, however, soon passed over. For some days he has felt completely well. No abnormal deposits in the urine. Appetite good. Treatment stopped to-day. He decided to let time and light injections cure the gleet.

The patient has had no trouble from his bladder since the above date.

Treatment.—The special treatment consisted of tapotement over the lower lumbar, sacral, and perineal regions; light shakings of the bladder, both from above the pubic arch and the perineum; vibrations above the pubic arch; nerve frictions for several minutes over the lower lumbar and the sacral nerves; and, lastly, pétrissage of the abdomen. The nerve frictions were the most effective in reducing the irritation and inflammation. The patient drank a considerable amount of water, acidulated with the fresh juice of lemons.

XXVI. MIGRAINE.

Mr. C. A., aged 27, had since August, 1888, suffered greatly from sudden onsets of violent headache. At first some time elapsed between each attack, but the intervals grew shorter until at length the patient had barely recovered from one attack before another began and in this manner more than a week would sometimes pass before he obtained complete relief.

The headaches are preceded by a heavy dull sensation in the head and shimmering (?) before the eyes in the morning when the patient awakes. The dull feeling passes away during the forenoon, but late in the afternoon pain suddenly sets in, and grows more and more severe toward night. The pain may reach its height at once, or its increase may be more gradual. It is throbbing in character, is felt most behind the eyes, and is generally equally acute on both sides. Light intensifies the pain. The patient dreads going to bed, because the recumbent position makes him worse. When he does lie

down, he after some hours goes off into a heavy sleep, and
wakes up the following morning with a feeling of oppressive
drowsiness, which on more than one occasion has lasted for
several days.

These attacks leave him very nervous and exhausted.

The patient never feels sick.

He has found that the headache is brought on by fatigue,
by sitting up at night, and by very strong light, as in theatres.

In the summer of 1888 he also became subject to attacks
of palpitation. The first rendered him nearly insensible; he
felt pain down his left arm, and had considerable difficulty in
drawing his breath.

During the attacks of palpitation, the apex beat is seen
and felt over a considerable area; the sounds are strong; the
pulse is between 80 and 90 beats a minute, and full. The
patient is very sensitive between the shoulders. The palpitation comes on at any time—sometimes it follows a meal,
sometimes several hours afterward.

The patient smokes cigarettes.

The appetite and digestion are good.

Treatment and Progress.—On the 4th January, 1890, he
was first subjected to treatment, which consisted of general
movements, and, as special applications for the migraine, frictions over the nerves of the head and neck; for the palpitation, nerve frictions between the shoulders and vibrations over
the apex of the heart.

At the end of January the attacks were less frequent, and
very often, although the premonitory symptoms appeared in
the morning, no headache followed, as treatment in the forenoon intervened. Palpitation has not occurred after the first
week of treatment. During this month the patient has been
treated regularly every day.

In the last week of February the treatment was discontinued, as there had been no headache for some time. When
they had come on they disappeared after a short application
of nerve frictions, alternating with pressure over the second
cervical pairs. The treatment had not been given regularly
during this month, often only two or three times a week. The
general condition has greatly improved; no palpitation during
the month.

10

XXVII. ACUTE INFLAMMATORY GASTRO-INTESTINAL CA-
TARRH IN A CHILD.

H. S., aged 15 months, was during the night of the 10th
July, 1889, suddenly seized with vomiting and diarrhœa. Up
till then he had been perfectly well. The stools grew more
frequent toward the morning, occurring every half-hour or
twenty minutes.

I first saw the child at 8 A.M. on the morning of the 11th
of July. The face had a pinched expression, the spaces round
the eyes were dark and sunken, the fontanelles depressed.
He was lying in a listless position, feebly whimpering every
now and then. The pulse was very feeble, and went at the
rate of 170 beats in the minute; the temperature was 102.2°.
The motions were watery, intermingled with little lumps and
some blood.

Treatment and Progress.—The local treatment consisted
of vibrations over the abdomen for about twenty-five minutes,
followed by slow and gentle pétrissage of the abdomen. Light
frictions over the dorsal nerves and those of the neck, and
some on the arms and legs, were also administered, partly
with a view to reducing the temperature and partly for
general stimulation.

When I returned in the afternoon at four o'clock, the
temperature had gone down to 100.6°; he had had four calls
to stool. The boy looked much better, he took notice of what
passed around him, and chattered all the time I treated him.

At eleven o'clock in the evening I found my patient peace-
fully asleep, having been in this condition for two hours. He
had been much better after I left in the afternoon.

July 12th, 4 P.M. The child had slept all through the
night; had no fever, no diarrhœa. Treatment same as day
before, and given for the last time. The boy was allowed to
rise the following day. Light and cautious diet was prescribed. There has been no relapse.

In September, 1886, I had also a patient, a boy ten years
old, suffering from the same complaint. He had turned ill
in the evening very suddenly when going to bed. The vomiting in this case was very distressing, the stools were more
watery, the pain in the abdomen was very considerable. I

treated him after the same manner as the above case. The sickness and diarrhœa ceased on the following morning.

XXVIII. Peritonitis.

A. S., aged 8, came under my care on July 13th, 1889. On the previous day he had complained of slight pain in the abdomen. The pain subsided toward the evening, but returned suddenly and with great violence on the following afternoon, accompanied by vomiting. I was at once sent for, but could not call before midnight. I then found the patient lying on his back with his knees drawn up, and the abdomen greatly distended. He complained of constant pain all over his abdomen, which was greatly increased by the slightest touch, movement of the body and legs, or by respiration. He was unable to draw his breath deeply; the respiration was short and thoracic. The pain was most intense in the epigastrium and round the umbilicus. There had been no action of the bowels. The temperature was 103°; pulse, 150.

Treatment and Progress.—After vibrations had been applied for about thirty minutes, the pain subsided to such an extent that the patient could stretch his legs out and could make deep respiration without much discomfort. I could now also make some pressure on the abdomen with the entire hand. Pointed touch with the fingers alone could not be endured. In addition to the vibrations, I gave frictions over the cervical nerves for several minutes, as well as over the dorsal sensory nerves.

July 14th. Forenoon. The boy had slept for about two hours after I left. He then woke up and became slightly delirious; the pain had also increased. Before leaving on my previous visit, I had shown the boy's mother what she had to do in case of a recurrence of the pain, and how she should apply the vibrations. She now made them at once, and the patient grew easier and slept again. Toward the morning he awoke once more, and for the second time she renewed the treatment, with good result. The temperature had fallen to 101°, the pulse to 120. The pain has considerably diminished, and the respiration is to a great extent abdominal. Treatment same as on my first visit. In the afternoon the temperature had fallen to 99.8°. Treatment repeated as before.

July 15th. I saw the patient in the afternoon. The temperature was normal; pressure only produced slight pain. Very light pétrissage of the abdomen was given for the first time. The patient could take a little fluid food, such as milk and beef-tea.

July 16th. The bowels were moved last night. Did not complain of pain. Treatment same as yesterday.

July 18th. The boy was allowed to get up and to lie dressed on the top of the bed. Could scarcely stand from weakness. Has had some finely-divided meat and fish. Bowels have been moved once a day.

July 22d. The patient has been up and about during the last three days. Treatment discontinued.

The vibrations served the purpose of relieving the pain, preventing peristalsis, and reducing the inflammation.

I should like to add that I feel greatly indebted to the boy's mother for the rapid progress toward recovery in the last two cases. She had herself for several years been more or less under manual treatment. She is gifted with an unusually good hand, and could therefore correctly apply the vibrations.

INDEX.

www.ingramcontent.com/pod-product-compliance
Lightning Source LLC
Chambersburg PA
CBHW021813190326
41518CB00007B/574